REALLY REAL YOGA © 1

YOUR NAME _____

With special thanks to the following students who helped make this manual exceptional.

Cover Chakra Illustration
Suzie Smith

Yoga Models
Alexis Kowitz
Amy Louise Williams
Dan Morgan
Diego Degiovanni
Elena Baracco
Francesca Clark
Gladys Duarte
Greta Grondahl
Hannah Strand
Jennifer Ohlsson
Jessie Hilgenberg
Kathleen Doyle
Kayla Hough
Megan Woodhall Carson
Rannveig Aamodt
Rolando Amorim

Author
Marianne Wells

Marianne Wells Yoga School is the longest running yoga school in Costa Rica.
Voted one of the top five destination yoga teacher trainings.
We offer seven yoga teacher trainings throughout the year.

www.mariannewells.com

Edition 2016.2
Publication Date: May 2016
Copyright © 2016 by Marianne Wells, LLC

IF MY HEART COULD DO MY THINKING

AND MY HEAD COULD TRULY FEEL

THEN I WOULD KNOW WHAT IS REALLY REAL

~ MARIANNE WELLS

#REALLYREALYOGA

GOD DOES NOT GIVE YOU WHAT YOU ASKED FOR

HE PROVIDES YOU WITH THE OPPORTUNITY

TO ACHIEVE IT ON YOUR OWN

~ EVAN ALMIGHTY

"You must begin from where you are." I begin every teacher training with these words. Beginning from where we are means accepting all of the things in our lives that we cannot change, and, acting upon those that we can. It is difficult to do for many – myself included – and takes years of practice.

I was not focused on yoga in my youth. I was raised in a family that incorporated a few aspects of Ayurveda and yoga into our daily routines, but, it was not a dominant theme of my upbringing. I developed a real, personal yoga practice after marriage and giving birth to my children in my early 20s. After moving to a new city, I was a stay-at-home mom who attended yoga classes in a church basement to socialize and make new friends. The teacher of that class became the woman that I call my yoga teacher. She was a student of B.K.S. Iyengar in a time when many people did not know what yoga was about, let alone who Iyengar was.

In the following years I earned a bachelor's degree in fine arts, and relocated once more to the Minneapolis area. Shortly after settling down in Minnesota, three things happened to me in rapid succession. Physically my body started to break down, largely due to my work as a muralist. Mentally, I was unfulfilled by the work. Spiritually, my grandfather passed away in my arms. Immediately following his passing, I shifted toward my Soul's true purpose on this Earth – teaching others. In a very short time, I was teaching yoga full-time across the Twin Cities. Yoga had been tapping me on the shoulder for a long time, but I had been focused on achieving other goals. This shift would be the start of a wonderfully positive era of service to others through the gifts of yoga.

I truly believe that when you find your Soul's purpose in this lifetime, it will be the easiest and most natural thing you do. Connecting with my students came naturally, and it was they who established the foundation of my philosophy – to teach people, not poses, by meeting people where they are. I always allowed my students to tell me what they wanted – to serve their needs. Through this deeply meaningful connection, my students gently took my hand as I had theirs. My devoted students helped to build my business. They spread my teaching around the Twin Cities, requested that I guide yoga retreats, and subqequently create a yoga teacher training. I listened closely to their need and in doing so, I have found tremendous fulfillment.

One of the first things that I teach in training is what I call Really Real Yoga. As yoga has become increasingly popular and commercialized, its true purpose has become muddled and neglected by some teachers. I believe my purpose, my Dharma, in this lifetime is to honor the lineage of yoga, and, to pass the ancient teachings of yoga on to my students. I believe my students' beginning should emerge from my lifetime of developing wisdom, focusing on the needs of the student, in service to others. I believe passionately in offering intensive teacher trainings because yoga – real yoga – is much more than asana. Yoga truly is a lifestyle; and, it is my purpose to pass the ancient wisdom of this way of life on to my students. As founder of the longest running yoga school in Costa Rica, I now have students in over 65 countries across the globe, and am recognized internationally as a leading destination yoga teacher training. Being a yoga teacher and running a yoga teacher training is not about the recognition or the money, though; it's simply about honoring real yoga and honoring those who honor us with their presence in each class. This is a sacred obligation in service and honor to others. Open. Honest. Heartfelt. Loving. That's why I always say, "If my heart could do my thinking, and my head could truly feel, then I would know what is really real."

In deep gratitude to this Universe for bringing beautiful Souls into my life, who have walked this path with me. ~ Marianne Wells

LOOK TO THIS DAY

FOR IT IS LIFE

THE VERY LIFE OF LIFE

IN ITS BRIEF COURSE LIE ALL

THE REALITIES AND VERITIES OF EXISTENCE

THE BLISS OF GROWTH

THE SPLENDOR OF ACTION

THE GLORY OF POWER

FOR YESTERDAY IS

BUT A DREAM

AND TOMORROW IS

ONLY A VISION

BUT TODAY

WELL LIVED

MAKES EVERY YESTERDAY

A DREAM OF HAPPINESS

AND EVERY TOMORROW

A VISION OF HOPE

LOOK WELL

THEREFORE TO THIS DAY

~ SANSKRIT PROVERB

CONTENTS

THERE ARE THREE THINGS EXTREMELY HARD

STEEL

A DIAMOND

AND TO KNOW ONE'S SELF

~ BENJAMIN FRANKLIN

YOUR BIOGRAPHY

BE, DON'T TRY TO BECOME. ~ OSHO

Write something about your family.

_____

Write something about your interests.

_____

Why are you passionate about yoga?

_____

Where do you like to travel?

_____

Why do you like to teach?

_____

What will students take away from your yoga classes?

_____

What is your teaching philosophy?

_____

List past jobs or careers:

_____

List your volunteer experience:

_____

List clubs or organizations you belong to:

_____

How did you connect to your mind, body and spirit as a child? As an adult? As you have aged?

_____

What form of yoga practice are you drawn to, and why?

_____

I AM ABOUT TO TREAD THE VERY SAME PATH

THAT HAS BEEN WALKED BY THE BUDDHA

AND BY HIS GREAT AND HOLY DISCIPLES

AN INDOLENT PERSON CANNOT FOLLOW THIS PATH

MAY MY ENERGY PREVAIL

MAY I SUCCEED

~ BHANTE HENEPOLA GUNARATANA

PERSONAL INTENTION

IF YOU DON'T GO WITHIN, YOU MIGHT GO WITHOUT. KNOWLEDGE BECOMES WISDOM WITH PRACTICE.

What is your favorite posture and why? _____
_____
_____

How does that posture help bring good health to your body? _____
_____
_____

How does that posture help bring good health to your mind? _____
_____
_____

How does that posture help bring good health to your Soul? _____
_____
_____

What is your purpose for attending this training experience, and why? _____
_____
_____

How does your goal interplay with the others with whom you are sharing this experience? _____
_____
_____

How can you bring your goal back into your life for the betterment of society? _____
_____
_____

What is your Soul's purpose for this lifetime? _____
_____
_____

How are you going to honor that purpose here on Earth? _____
_____
_____

FOLLOW THAT ADVICE OF MINE WHICH IS GOOD

AND HELPFUL FOR YOUR PROGRESS

AND NEGLECT EVEN MY OWN ADVICE

WHICH IS NOT

~ UPANISHADS

LEARNING STYLE TEST

TO LEARN, READ. TO KNOW, WRITE. TO MASTER, TEACH.

Rank the words below. For each row across numbered 1-9, you will give a 4 to the words that best characterize your learning style, a 3 to the next best, a 2 to the next, a 1 to the words that least characterize your learning style. Be sure to use the numbers "1, 2, 3, 4" with each set of words.

1) _____ discriminating	_____ tentative	_____ involved	_____ practical
2) _____ receptive	_____ relevant	_____ analytical	_____ impartial
3) _____ feeling	_____ watching	_____ thinking	_____ doing
4) _____ accepting	_____ risk-taker	_____ evaluative	_____ aware
5) _____ intuitive	_____ productive	_____ logical	_____ questioning
6) _____ abstract	_____ observing	_____ concrete	_____ active
7) _____ present-oriented	_____ reflecting	_____ future-oriented	_____ pragmatic
8) _____ experience	_____ observation	_____ conceptualization	_____ experimental
9) _____ intense	_____ reserved	_____ rational	_____ responsible

add lines 2 3 4 5 7 8

A_____

add lines 1 3 6 7 8 9

B_____

add lines 2 3 4 5 8 9

C_____

add lines 1 3 6 7 8 9

D_____

A Concrete Experience

(doer)

D Active Experimentation

(feeler)

B Reflective Observation

(watcher)

C Abstract Conceptualization

(thinker)

Yoga Philosophy and Your Life

Yoga is best known in the West for the physical nature of the asana practices. As one progresses in their yoga practice, there is a great possibility that other aspects open up to them. A sense of calm. Peacefulness. Insight into how one is living their life. And seeing oneself in others – at least to some extent in a few aspects of living.

In my opinion, what keeps yoga relevant to society as the generations pass by is less about the physical practice – the physical body – and more about how yoga impacts the more subtle levels of our existence. Of course, as humans in this body, we must progress through the physical layer. It's why Pattabhi Jois said, "Do your practice. All will come." He was referring to the realization of these deeper levels, but much more than just the Ashtanga asana series and pranayama. These are techniques or gateways to deeper understanding.

I believe that any serious study of yoga must begin with the philosophy of yoga. Yoga is a psychological method of self-controlling the thought processes of our minds. This is not brainwashing by any means, but a way of progression in self-awareness and self-understanding. Once we know ourselves well, we learn the lessons of our lives. We learn to get out of our own way when necessary. In taking the time to understand ourselves, we gain a deeper awareness of the world around us – especially the people that we interact with on a frequent basis. We develop a greater tolerance for others. We seek out the counterpoint to our positions. We become less reactive, as what was formerly viewed to be oppositional, competitive, or even threatening, now becomes one part of the greater picture. We are inclusive.

The Yoga Sutras of Patanjali are universal in the approach to living a good life. Written well before the genesis of the great religions of today, the Sutras share a common thread of how to treat yourself and others.

We share every word of the Yoga Sutras in our training in a communal setting – sharing what it means, processed through our students' personal lenses. The Sutras teach us that in yoga – and in life – direction is more important than force. It all comes out on the mat in our physical practice. As we advance, we become more quiet, more subtle. This reflects in our understanding and nurturing of our subtle bodies – the Kosha bodies. While not a theistic belief system per se, yoga does tend to open channels through our energy layers to at least briefly experience the spiritual nature into which we were born and, ultimately, pass from this level of existence.

We come to understand the levels of human consciousness. In understanding that direction is more important than force, we understand there is an important aspect to the energy that we project and attract. We become very mindful of our personal narrative – how do we think about ourselves and how do we communicate this to others? Our thoughts become our words which motivate actions. Understanding the process of the mind is a powerful key to this enlightening direction in life. It allows for both change and acceptance in very powerful ways.

All energy moves toward the ultimate thresholds of human consciousness – Love, Joy, Peace. We feel these levels for brief and even prolonged moments in our lives. Yoga helps us to understand how to cultivate this, but not as a direct goal because that becomes a desire which can often frustrate. You can't yell at someone – "Love me!" – and have it be so. It is more an outcome of doing the things in life that lead to less complication, less self-interest, toward serving the needs of others in a way that works within our own personal Dharma. My Dharma happens to be teaching yoga in a way that emphasizes a respect for this process.

This area of study and understanding provides a yoga teacher with a very rich resource of teaching to others. Study of the philosophy of yoga can help provide a foundation for living life with purpose, with intention. Intention sets forth the thoughts and actions that follow. While people come to yoga for many things, ultimately it is to be calm with less stress and a greater understanding of themselves and the greater whole. Study of philosophy is often our students' favorite part of teacher training because it helps find some answers to their life questions. Really Real Yoga helps to illuminate your Soul's real purpose in this life. In other words, how do your gifts meet the world's needs?

THE MOST BASIC AIM OF YOGA

TO AWAKEN MENTALLY BY LOOKING INSIDE OURSELVES

TO USE THIS AWAKENING TO OVERCOME OUR LIMITATIONS

AND TO UNDERSTAND, ACCEPT AND LIVE, TRULY THINK POSITIVELY

~ UNKNOWN

PUT YOUR HEART, MIND, INTELLECT AND SOUL

INTO YOUR SMALLEST ACTS

THIS IS THE SECRET OF SUCCESS

~ SWAMI SIVANANDA

THE YOGA SUTRAS OF PATANJALI — CHAPTER ONE

BEFORE WE CAN SEE TO LEARN, WE MUST FIRST LEARN TO SEE ~ JOE K.

What is Yoga

1 Now the teaching of yoga are steps that allow one to progress.

2 Yoga is the ability to direct and focus mental activity and the ability to still the turning of thought.

3 With attainment of a focused mind — pure awareness — the inner being spirit stands in its true identity observing the world.

4 Otherwise, the observer identifies with the turning of thought, the activities of the mind.

What is the Mind and the Turning of Thought

5 There are five activities of the mind, including both suffering and non-suffering.

6 The five mental activities are — understanding, error, conceptualization, deep sleep and memory.

7 Understanding arises from sensory perception, inference and the faithful words of others.

8 Error is false knowledge based on misinterpretation of reality.

9 Conceptualization is based on words that are not connected with real things.

10 Deep sleep is the turning of thought abstracted from existence.

11 Memory is the recollection of objects one has experienced.

Practice and Dispassion

12 Both practice and non-reaction are required to still the turning of thought.

13 Practice is the effort to attain cessation of thought, creating stillness as a state of mental peace.

14 This practice is firmly rooted only when it is cultivated with respect and skill for a long uninterrupted period.

15 Non-reaction is mastery over the desire for sensuous objects, whether perceived directly or learned.

16 When non-reaction has been reached, one has no desire for anything material because of the conscious spiritual principle.

Ways of Stopping Thought

17 Full conscious and pure contemplation are accompanied by four kinds of processes of knowing: analytical thinking, insight, bliss and feeling like self.

18 Later, after one practices steadily to bring thought to a standstill, these four kinds of thought fall away and only sublimated impressions remain.

19 These impressions are innate for two kinds of beings — Those without a body and those who are reabsorbed into original matter.

20 For the others, faith, energy, mindfulness, contemplative calm and wisdom form the path to realization.

21 For those who seek liberation wholeheartedly, the goal of realization is near.

22 How near depends on whether the practice is mild, moderate or intense.

Dedication to the Lord of Yoga – God – Isvara

23 Realization may also come if one is oriented toward the idea of pure awareness and devotion to the Divine.

24 Isvara contains the form of pure awareness, independent of corruption from actions and consequences of persons.

25 Isvara is the incomparable seed of omniscience.

26 Being unconditioned by time, Isvara is the spiritual teacher of even the ancient teachers.

27 Isvara is represented by the sacred syllable AUM, the sound OM.

28 Repeating AUM and pondering its meaning leads to understanding, overcoming obstacles and distractions.

29 With AUM, self-understanding is attained and obstacles fall away.

30 The obstacles that distract the mind are sickness, lack of emotion, doubt, carelessness, laziness, sexual indulgence, delusion, lack of progress and restlessness. These all act as barriers to stillness.

31 These distractions can cause suffering and depression, interfering with steady breath and posture.

32 The practice of focusing on a single truth or one of the principals of yoga keeps these obstacles at a distance.

Tranquility of Thought

33 The mind becomes quiet and consciousness settles as one cultivates friendship, compassion, joy, evenness of mind toward all things, whether pleasant or painful, good or bad.

34 Or the mind becomes quiet and serene through prolonged exhalation and holding of breath.

35 Or the mind becomes quiet and serene through steady observation of sensory input.

36 Or the mind becomes quiet and serene when thoughts are luminous and free from sorrow.

37 Or the mind becomes quiet and serene by focusing on things that do not inspire attachment.

38 Or the mind becomes quiet and serene through reflections from dreams and sleep.

39 Or the mind becomes quiet and serene through meditation on a suitable object.

40 When the mind is quiet and serene thought is tranquil, it extends to the infinite, both small and vast.

Contemplation That Bears Seeds, Bringing You to the Next Level

41 As pattern of thought subsides, a transparent way of "seeing" becomes clear and comes together. Like a jewel, this seeing will reflect equally whatever lies before it, whether people, object or thoughts.

42 So long as contemplation is transparent and you can look past preconceptions, then you can see the essence for all that it truly is.

43 Beyond transparent contemplation, memory is purified and you understand clearly.

44 Such contemplation intuitively grasps subtle objects in their reality and beyond.

45 The ability to see the subtlety of objects is dependent on your ability to perceive the object.

46 These four stages – 41 to 44 – are required to bear seeds.

Seedless Contemplation, Thought Ceases, Spirit is Free From the Material World

47 Once you master contemplation, the essence of the Self becomes clear. Bringing tranquility, stillness, clarity, serenity and inner peace. Only now can you truly begin to know yourself in this world.

48 Wisdom acquired from contemplation is an automatic way of seeing absolute truth, leading to knowledge.

49 Wisdom acquired is non-mental and knowledge is acquired without thought. The thinking mind no longer gets in the way. Yoga emphasizes this direct relationship. If you can perceive an object, you can know an object and you don't have to think about that object.

50 The impressions generated by wisdom prevent other formations of impressions.

51 When the turning of thought ceases completely, seedless contemplation appears.

LET US BOW BEFORE THE NOBLEST OF SAGES PATANJALI

WHO GAVE YOGA FOR SERENITY

AND SANCTITY OF MIND

GRAMMAR FOR CLARITY AND PURITY OF SPEECH

AND MEDICINE FOR PERFECTION OF HEALTH

LET US PROSTRATE BEFORE PATANJALI

AN INCARNATION OF ADISESA

WHOSE UPPER BODY HAS A HUMAN FORM

WHOSE ARMS HOLD A CONCH AND A DISC

AND WHO IS CROWNED BY A THOUSAND-HEADED COBRA

~ IYENGAR INVOCATION HONORING PATANJALI

SELF-STUDY QUIZ

Please explain Yoga Sutra 1.12 (hint, the present moment and letting go):

_____

_____

_____

_____

How exactly does Yoga Sutra 1.13 teach persevering practice?

_____

_____

_____

_____

Yoga Sutra 1.22 teaches about temperament, what temperament is that Sutra referring to?

_____

_____

_____

_____

Please explain how Yoga Sutra 1.23 allows for all to practice within their personal faith.

_____

_____

_____

_____

In Sutra 1.51, what is meant by seedless contemplation? Please refer to Sutras in Chapter 1.

_____

_____

_____

_____

SELF-STUDY QUIZ

Based on Chapter 1 of the Yoga Sutras, Patanjali states that, "yoga is a method of bringing consciousness to a state of stillness." In the space below, please elaborate as this statement applies to you.

_____
_____
_____
_____

Based on Chapter 1 of the Yoga Sutras, Patanjali lays out how to calm the mind. In the space below please elaborate how this statement applies to you, and how you can apply this thought to a class you are teaching.

_____
_____
_____
_____

How does suffering end?

_____
_____
_____
_____

In a yoga practice, one looks inside to learn about themselves. How does this happen?

_____
_____
_____

Who or what are the "Upanishads?"

_____
_____
_____
_____

THE YOGA SUTRAS OF PATANJALI — CHAPTER TWO

THE PURPOSE OF YOGA IS; DISCIPLINE, SELF-STUDY, SURRENDER

The Purpose of Yoga

1 The active performance of yoga involves three components – discipline, self-study of sacred texts, and surrendering to pure awareness.

2 Its purpose is to – one – cultivate pure contemplation and – two – diminish the causes of suffering.

Definition of the Forces of Corruption

3 The causes of suffering are – ignorance (or not seeing things as they are), "I" ego, attachment, hatred or aversion or repulsion, and the will to live or clinging to life out of fear of death.

4 Ignorance, or not seeing things as they are, is the field that initiates the other four causes of suffering whether they are dormant, weakened, intermittent or active.

5 Ignorance is the confusion of the temporary with the permanent, the pure with the impure, the pleasure in suffering or the anguish with the pleasure of being, the relative with the absolute or the essential Self where there is no Self.

6 Ego "I" ascribes to mental and physical activity as the source of consciousness, a unified self in pure awareness. The power to see – "before we can see to learn, we must first learn to see."

7 Attachment is the residue or consequence of pleasurable experiences.

8 Aversion is the residue or consequence of suffering or displeasure.

9 The will to live is instinctive and self-perpetuating, even for the learned sage.

Removing the Forces of Corruption

10 In their subtle form, these causes of suffering are subdued by seeing where they come from.

11 One can escape the effect of their turnings through meditative absorption.

12 Acts stemming from mental disturbance leave imprints that always show themselves in some form or another. All actions deposit latent impressions deep in the mind to be activated in this birth or a future one.

13 As long as this root source exists, its contents will ripen into a birth, a life and experience in the world.

14 These actions bear joyful or sorrowful fruits in proportion to good or bad actions that are stored latent impressions.

15 The wise man sees all that as suffering because of the sufferings inherent in change and its corrupting subliminal impressions and because of the way qualities of material nature turn against themselves.

16 Suffering that has not come yet can be prevented or escaped.

What are the Two Levels of Being – the Observer and the Phenomenal World

17 The cause of suffering is the connection between the observer and the phenomenal world.

18 The phenomenal world has clarity, activity and inertia, and is made up of the elements and the senses. This world can serve the goals of sensual experience and spiritual liberation.

19 The origin and characteristics of things are structured as specific, nonspecific, marked and unmarked.

20 Pure awareness is just seeing itself; although pure, it usually appears to operate through the perceiving mind.

21 In essence, the phenomenal world exists only in relation to an observer.

22 Once this happens, the phenomenal world no longer appears as such, though it continues to exist as a common reality for everyone else.

23 It is by virtue of the apparent indivisibility of awareness and the phenomenal world that permits understanding of their respective faculties.

24 The cause of this union is ignorance.

25 When there is no ignorance, there is no such connection – the freedom of the observer lies in its absence.

26 The way to eliminate ignorance is through steady, focused discrimination between the observer and the world.

27 The ultimate wisdom that emerges has seven stages. How do the eight limbs help me attain the yoga state?

The Limbs of the Yoga Practice

28 When impurity is destroyed by practicing the limbs of yoga, the light of knowledge shines in focus.

29 The eight limbs of yoga are – moral principles, observances, posture, breath control, withdrawal of the senses, concentration, meditation and pure contemplation.

The Moral Principles and Observances

30 The universal moral principles are — nonviolence, truth, avoid stealing, celibacy, absence of greed.

31 These universal moral principles, unrestricted by birth, place, era or circumstance, are the great vow of yoga.

32 The five internal disciplines are bodily purification, contentment, a disciplined life, study of sacred texts, dedication to Isvara, the Lord of yoga.

33 Unwholesome thoughts can be neutralized by cultivating wholesome ones.

34 Unwholesome thoughts may arise from greed, anger or delusion and they will cause suffering and ignorance.

The Moral Principles

35 Being firmly grounded in nonviolence creates an atmosphere in which others can let go of their hostility.

36 For one grounded in truthfulness, every action and its result are grounded in truth.

37 All the jewels appear for one who is firmly set in honesty.

38 Vitality appears in one who is firmly set in moderation.

39 When one is without greed, the riddle of rebirth is revealed.

The Observances

40 With bodily purification, one's body ceases to be compelling and non-physical relationships emerge.

41 Purification also brings clarity, mental happiness, psychic focus, mastery of the senses, self-awareness.

42 Contentment brings supreme happiness.

43 Perfection of the body and senses come from practice, which destroys impurities.

44 Communion with one's chosen deity comes from the study of sacred lore.

45 The perfection of pure contemplation comes from dedication to the Lord of Yoga.

Posture

46 The posture of yoga is steady and easy, firm and soft.

47 It is realized by relaxing one's effort and resting like the cosmic serpent on the waters of infinity.

48 Then one is no longer disturbed by the play of opposites.

Breath Control

49 When the posture is steady, then breath control is the regulation of exhalation and inhalation.

50 As one observes the phases of the breath in space, time and number, the breath becomes spacious and subtle.

51 A fourth type of breath control goes beyond the range of exhalation and inhalation.

52 The veil that covers the light of truth dissolves.

53 And the mind is now fit for concentration.

Withdrawal of the Senses

54 Withdrawal of the senses occurs when the sensory organs are independent of their particular objects.

55 From this comes complete control of the senses.

SELF-STUDY QUIZ

Yoga Sutras 2.1 and 2.2 talk about the purpose of yoga. Based on Sutras 2.3 – 2.16, keep these two words in mind – attachment and aversion. With these words in mind, what obstacles do our personalities present?

_____

_____

_____

_____

How do we perceive the world around us? (Refer to Yoga Sutra 2.19)

_____

_____

_____

_____

How do Yoga Sutras 2.28 and 2.29 prepare us for teachings of the eight limbs?

_____

_____

_____

_____

Elaborate on how the yamas in Yoga Sutra 2.30 are listed in order of priority.

_____

_____

_____

_____

Elaborate on how the niyamas in Yoga Sutra 2.32 are independent of each other.

_____

_____

_____

_____

SELF-STUDY QUIZ

How can a posture be both firm and soft? Please quote from the Yoga Sutras, particularly Sutra 2.46, and from class.

_____

_____

_____

_____

How does your breath become fit for concentration? Please quote from Yoga Sutras, particularly Sutra 2.53, and from class.

_____

_____

_____

_____

How are the senses perfectly mastered? Please quote from the Yoga Sutras, particularly Sutra 2.55, and from class.

_____

_____

_____

_____

Yoga is a method of bringing consciousness to a state of stillness. How do we find motion and stillness? How do we find effort and effortlessness?

_____

_____

_____

_____

According to Patanjali and others, the ignorance of one's truth is the root cause of suffering. What is truth and how do we arrive at a rational conclusion on the question of truth?

_____

_____

_____

_____

THE YOGA SUTRAS OF PATANJALI — CHAPTER THREE

ACT LIKE THE PERSON YOU WANT TO BE

What are the Steps Toward Mastery – Perfect Discipline

1 Concentration is binding thought in one place.

2 Meditative absorption is focusing on a single conceptual flow.

3 When the essential nature of the object shines forth, as if formless, integration of meditation is concentration.

What is Mastery – Perfect Discipline and how do We use it?

4 Concentration, meditation and pure contemplation, focused on a single object, constitute perfect discipline.

5 The light of wisdom comes from mastery of perfect discipline.

6 The practice of perfect discipline is achieved in stages.

7 Of the eight limbs, the last three — concentration, meditation and integration — are more internal than the preceding five.

8 Even these three are external limbs of integration that bears no seeds.

What are the Different Stages of Transformation

9 Transformation toward total stillness occurs when latent impressions arise, mental distractions are overcome and stillness emerges in its place.

10 These latent impressions help consciousness flow from one tranquil moment to the next.

11 The transformation of thought toward pure contemplation occurs when distractions vanish and the mind becomes focused.

12 Transformation of thought toward psychic focus occurs between a rest and arising state.

What do We Mean by Exceptional Faculties

13 The evolution of thought explains the fundamental tendencies — relationship of time, nature's physical state, and physical condition, all of which occur in material elements and the organs.

14 One substratum underlying the properties of nature contain past, present and future characteristics.

15 Different methods produce different changes.

Exceptional Faculties – the Powers of Extraordinary Knowledge

16 Knowledge of the past and the future comes from perfect discipline of the three transformations of thought — fundamental, temporal and situational.

17 Confusion arises from the interaction of words, objects and ideas with one another. The perfect distinction between them allows knowledge and understanding of the language of all beings.

18 Knowledge about the origins of former births appear when we gain insight into our own conditioning.

19 Knowing what another is thinking comes from focusing with perfect discipline on the perceptions of another.

20 The knowledge of another's thought does not yield insight because the object itself is not actually present in that person's consciousness.

Exceptional Faculties – the Powers of Perfect Discipline

21 When the body has perfect discipline, it becomes invisible, allowing one to disassociate the observer's gaze and blocking the contact of light from one's eyes.

22 Perfect discipline of the slow and rapid effects of action brings knowledge of the time and circumstances of one's death. Also known as premonition.

23 Perfect discipline of friendship, compassion, joy and impartiality confers corresponding power.

24 By perfect concentration on the strength of an animal, such as the elephant, one gains their strength.

25 From placing light on the mind, one has knowledge and insight on the subtle, hidden and distant.

26 Perfect concentration on the sun bestows knowledge of the universe.

27 Perfect concentration on the moon bestows knowledge of star positions.

28 Perfect concentration on the polestar bestows knowledge of the movement of the stars.

29 Perfect concentration on the energy center of the navel yields knowledge of the body and its physiology.

30 Perfect discipline on the throat frees one from hunger and thirst.

31 Perfect discipline on the "tortoise channel" brings steadiness.

32 Perfect concentration on the light on the top of the head brings visions of perfected beings.

33 Through intuition, all is known.

34 Perfect concentration on the heart reveals the contents of one's thoughts.

35 The spirit is different from steady withdrawing of the senses. From perfect discipline of the spirit, one gains knowledge.

36 From this knowledge appears intuitive forms of hearing, touch, clairvoyance, taste and sensitive sense of smell.

What Dangers do They Present

37 If these faculties become a distraction, these powers of perfection are impediments to pure contemplation.

What are These Exceptional Faculties – Mastery of the Physical World

38 By relaxing one's attachment to the body and from awareness of the body's currents, one can influence another's mind and body.

39 With perfect mastery of the flow of energy in the head and neck, one rises above water, mud and thorns.

40 Perfect mastery of the flow of energy through the solar plexus, one acquires a fiery radiance.

41 Perfect mastery of the relationship between the ear and space, one has divine hearing.

42 Mastering the relationship between the body and ether, then meditating on the lightness of cotton, one can move through space.

43 When outside things no longer condition mental activity, called "The Great Disembodied Thought," the veil that obscures the light is destroyed.

44 Mastering the gross, subtle, intrinsic and purposive brings mastery of the five elements.

45 Perfect mastery of the five elements brings mastery of physical form, physical vigor and freedom from physical constraint.

Other Powers

46 Bodily perfection consists of physical beauty, charm – grace, strength and being as solid as a diamond.

47 From perfect discipline of perception, intrinsic natures, relational and purposes brings mastery of the organs.

48 From this, one acquires instantaneous thought, perception without the aid of the senses, and perfect mastery of origins appear.

49 Complete revelation of the difference between pure awareness and the luminous aspect of the phenomenal world, all conditions are known and mastered.

The Limitations of These Powers – What Should We Avoid

50 Spiritual liberation comes when one is unattached to this omniscience and the seeds of sin are destroyed.

51 One should avoid enthusiasm or pride in the enticements of the gods or suffering will recur.

The Limitations of These Powers – What is Ultimate Realization

52 Perfect mastery of moments and their sequence in time brings knowledge born of highly distinctive perception.

53 This specific knowledge allows comprehension of different origins, characteristics or situations that distinguish two seemingly similar things.

54 Knowledge born of discrimination flows spontaneously and pertains to all states of things at any level.

55 Absolute freedom occurs when the purity of the peaceful mind is identical (or in pure equilibrium) with that of the spiritual entity.

SELF-STUDY QUIZ

Based on Yoga Sutras 3.1 - 3.8, what are the steps toward mastery?

_____

_____

_____

_____

Based on Yoga Sutras 3.9 - 3.12, what are the different stages of transformation?

_____

_____

_____

_____

Based on Yoga Sutras 3.13 - 3.36, what do we mean by exceptional faculties?

_____

_____

_____

_____

Refer to Yoga Sutra 3.40 and discuss vital energy in the navel area.

_____

_____

_____

_____

Refer to Yoga Sutra 3.40 and discuss refinement of the senses.

_____

_____

_____

_____

SELF-STUDY QUIZ

Based on Chapter 3, what dangers do the exceptional faculties present?

_____

_____

_____

_____

Based on Chapter 3, according to Patanjali, what is the method to reach ultimate realization?

_____

_____

_____

_____

Based on Chapter 3, what should we avoid?

_____

_____

_____

_____

How do the eight limbs help one attain the yoga state?

_____

_____

_____

_____

Senses bring information into the body. How do we quiet the senses based on the eight limbs?

_____

_____

_____

_____

THE YOGA SUTRAS OF PATANJALI — CHAPTER FOUR

THE ONLY THING WE CANNOT CHANGE IS THE DAY WE WERE BORN, THE PARENTS WE WERE BORN TO,
AND THE DAY WE ARE GOING TO DIE

Where do Exceptional Faculties Come From
1 Powers of perfection arise from birth, through the use of herbs, spells — mantras, ascetic discipline and contemplation.

What is the Human Psyche
2 Positive transformation is the result of one's innermost nature.
3 The causes of transformation do not set nature in motion, but withdraw, like a gardener opening an irrigation canal.

The Transformation of Thought
4 Individual thoughts develop from a measure of egoism.
5 A single thought is operative over many others in diverse activities.
6 A thought which arises from meditation produces no negative influence over others.

The Transformation of Action
7 The yogi's actions are neither black nor white; the actions of others are black or white or both.
8 Consequences surely follow these inappropriate tendencies.
9 Despite differences in birth, place and time, the continuity of subliminal impressions is sustained because of the uniformity of memory.
10 These subliminal impressions are without beginning because the desire for life is eternal.
11 Cause, effect, bases and object are interdependent and when they cease to exist, the impressions also cease to exist.

The Reality of Material Things and the Structure of Thought
12 The past and future are always potentially present because the properties of nature move at different tempos.
13 The characteristics of these sectors, whether manifest or subtle, depends on the three qualities of nature.
14 An object's reality depends on uniting the transformation of the three constituent qualities of nature.
15 People perceive the same object differently, as each person's perception follows a separate path from another's.
16 For an object to exist, the mind need not perceive it. Without perception will it still exist, even though unknown?
17 The mind will or will not perceive an object depending on the attraction it exerts or the interest one has in it.

Thought and Spirit
18 The spirit never subjects to change, always knows, and is master of the turning of thought.
19 Since thought is an object of perception, it cannot illuminate itself.
20 And it is impossible for thought and its object to be comprehended simultaneously.
21 If a thought is the object of another thought, there is an infinite regression of phenomena and a confusion of memory.
22 When the mind is not turned outward, it reflects consciousness itself.

Thought and the Observer
23 Colored by both the observer and the phenomenal world, the mind can take everything as its object.
24 Although diversified by countless latent traits, thought works by making associations on behalf of a higher entity to serve awareness.
25 One who can distinguish between consciousness and awareness is freed from all searching for the inner being.
26 Then the mind is in deep discrimination and thought can gravitate toward freedom.

What can We do if We Lose This State of Liberation

27 When discernment lapses, distracting thoughts emerge from the store of latent impressions.

28 These distracting thoughts can be eliminated by tracing them back to their origin and by meditation.

29 For one who seeks no gain in vast knowledge, regardless of time, place or circumstance, one enters the final stage of integration called the essential cloud of virtuous harmony.

30 On account of this, all forces of corruption and action have vanished.

The Knowledge That Ends in Freedom

31 Then knowledge is more or less infinite, all the layers of imperfections concealing truth have been washed away, and little remains to be known.

32 This infinite knowledge means an end to the sequence of transformations in material things, their purpose now fulfilled.

33 The succession of moments appears as a series of events, each corresponding to the merest interest of time, in which one moment is correlative to the next moment.

34 Freedom is at hand when the fundamental qualities of nature are no longer a source of meaning or interest to the spiritual entities. Freedom is the power of consciousness founded in a state of true identity. That is all.

ACCORDING TO PATANJALI, YOGA IS THE CONTROL OF THE MIND.

HE REALIZED THAT ONE'S MIND CAN LEAD THEM INTO BONDAGE OR INTO LIBERATION.

MOST HUMAN PROBLEMS ORIGINATE IN THE MIND.

AND THE ONLY REMEDY IS MENTAL DISCIPLINE.

MANY MEDICAL EXPERTS AGREE THAT THE MAJORITY OF DISEASES ARE PSYCHOSOMATIC.

IF WE LEARN YOGA PHILOSOPHY AND TRULY ABSORB ITS ESSENCE,

WE CAN TAP INTO THE 90% OF OUR BRAINS THAT ARE NOW UNTOUCHED.

YOGA TEACHES US TO LOOK INSIDE OURSELVES, OUR MINDS,

OUR BODIES AND OUR HEARTS FOR CLUES AND ANSWERS.

YOGA GIVES US THE TOOLS NEEDED TO OVERCOME THE LIMITATIONS OF OUR SELVES.

WHEN YOU ARE INSPIRED BY SOME GREAT PURPOSE, SOME EXTRAORDINARY PROJECT,

ALL YOUR THOUGHTS BREAK THEIR BONDS. YOUR MIND TRANSCENDS LIMITATIONS,

YOUR CONSCIOUSNESS EXPANDS IN EVERY DIRECTION AND

YOU FIND YOURSELF IN A NEW, GREAT AND WONDERFUL WORLD.

DORMANT FORCES, FACULTIES AND TALENTS BECOME ALIVE,

AND YOU DISCOVER YOURSELF TO BE

A GREATER PERSON BY FAR THAN YOU EVER DREAMED YOURSELF TO BE.

~ PATANJALI

SELF-STUDY QUIZ

What is the foundation of your breath?

_____

_____

_____

Which pose is the most important first step in meditation?

_____

_____

_____

How can we find our essential nature of our being, and how does it apply to the universe?

_____

_____

_____

How will you help others understand that yoga is much more than a form of physical exercise?

_____

_____

_____

If a student, even after months of yoga, still cannot relax, what could you do to help them achieve this state?

_____

_____

_____

Why are inversions so good for you?

_____

_____

_____

Inversions should not be practiced by those with which conditions? List all you can remember.

_____

_____

_____

SELF-STUDY QUIZ

Where does the Spirit reside?

_____

_____

_____

What is the path to inner peace?

_____

_____

_____

The center of the physical body is the _____. All yoga postures originate from _____.
Teach a pose (or a few postures) from both the center and the origination points.

_____

_____

_____

Yoga is over 5,000 years old and was introduced to the United States more than 100 years ago.
Why then is yoga just now becoming so popular?

_____

_____

_____

The physical body is born, grows, changes, decays and then dies. How many other "bodies" are
attached to the physical body? How do these bodies affect the physical body?

_____

_____

_____

What are the guidelines for physical actions as long as we live in a physical body?

_____

_____

_____

Yoga and Ayurveda

Sister sciences that evolved in India, the relationship of yoga and Ayurveda go back in history for thousands of years. While yoga is more of a psychological method of stilling the mind, Ayurveda involves living in harmony with our natural constitution and the world around us.

Yoga is the deeper study of the Self. Yoga allows for Self-realization in reaching higher levels of consciousness, shedding the confines of the ego and realizing that we are all part of a greater whole of existence.

One of the main tenets of Ayurveda is that when we live in balance, in harmony with our natural constitution, we live with ease. Disease occurs when we are out of balance – through diet, lifestyle, environment, etc. Ayurveda provides an understanding of our fundamental tendencies – physically, emotionally, energetically and socially. I believe that many of the corporate interpersonal communication – relationship programs such as I-Speak, Meyers-Briggs, etc., can trace their evolution to Ayurveda. Knowing what our tendencies are, and recognizing the tendencies in others, provide a basis for how we and others relate to the world around us. It allows for greater understanding of why people react to certain stimuli, foods, situations, different times of day.

Wired into our DNA is how we look and, at a deeper level, behave. Ayurveda can help explain why siblings with the same parents can look and act very differently. One may be tall and thin with dry skin, the other may be heavier with lustrous complexion and thick, shiny hair. Ayurveda can provide an understanding of why certain individuals tend to be sluggish in the morning, or quick to anger when things don't go their way, or hard to understand because they can't focus on the moment at hand. This deeper understanding provides a basis of cooperation, of acceptance for being a unique individual. We learn to work together based on our strengths, not our differences.

In yoga, the diet is fairly simple – don't eat animals. Eating animals is a form of violence and increases the tamasic quality (makes us sluggish). Knowing how to eat the yoga way is illumination. In Ayurveda, it is important to recognize the food tastes that soothe our particular dosha (how we are made) and which ones can aggravate it. Even though there are activities and foods that we love, we learn to balance what we desire with what's best for us.

Ayurveda is self-healing; a healthy self-care way of living every day. Once we realize that we become what we eat and how we live, we are empowered to be mindful in the choices that we make every single day. Knowing how to eat the Ayurveda way is healing, balanced, satisfying to our systems.

By this logic Ayurveda should be more popular than yoga. I am surprised that more people don't know more about Ayurveda. We talk a great deal about food in Ayurveda, as food is life. The very building blocks of our bodies are formed by what we consume each day, in food, drink and thoughts. Ayurveda changes our relationship to food and life quality. In my opinion, Ayurveda is an essential part of maintaining a healthy body and mind, freeing us to actively explore the deeper wonders of yoga.

Come explore the wonders of Ayurveda! As a yoga practitioner, Ayurveda provides a deeper level of understanding in how to live more mindfully and, as an individual, in being honest with ourselves at all times in the choices we make and don't make. As a yoga teacher, Ayurveda can provide an understanding of the tendencies that students bring to you each day. How we as teachers meet our students on their levels is vital to teaching people, not poses.

TEACHERS MUST HAVE PROPER TRAINING

MUST ALLOW FOR PROPER WARM-UP

MUST LOOK FOR PROPER POSTURE ALIGNMENT

AND MUST EDUCATE THEIR STUDENTS ON A HEALTHY LIFESTYLE

THAT INCLUDES CHANGES

CONSIDER H.A.L.T.

NEVER GET TOO HUNGRY

KNOW WHAT A QUALITY DIET IS

NEVER GET TOO ANGRY

TAKE TIME FOR MINDFUL RELAXATION

NEVER GET TOO LONELY

REDUCE TOXIC HABITS

NEVER GET TOO TIRED

DO YOUR DAILY YOGA THERAPY

THAT INCLUDES BREATH EXERCISES

UNDERSTANDING AYURVEDA

TO TAKE CARE OF OUR BODIES AND OUR LIFE WE NEED TO ADDRESS ALL THREE LEVELS. INCLUDING, SURRENDER, DEVOTION, AND APPLIED PHILOSOPHY. ~ T. KRISHNAMACHARYA

Ayurvedic living is a sacred, holistic life-science passed down from countless generations of Indian healers to the modern world by embracing and bringing together the mind, actions, body, environment and spirituality. This ancient science dates to at least the Vedic period, if not earlier, and at its core is the enduring belief that health exists when the tri-doshas – vata, kapha and pitta – are in balance. Ayurveda, itself, is derived from ayn "life" and veda "knowing."

Ayurvedic philosophy postulates a holistic understanding that energy and matter are one and that the five basic elements – space, air, fire, water and earth – come together within the body to form the tridoshas – vata, kapha and pitta. Vata (wind) is comprised of air and ether; kapha (moon) consists of earth and water, and pitta (sun) is composed of fire and earth.

Each dosha has certain fundamental characteristics which make it unique:

• Vata is associated with air, respiration, movement of bowels, bladder, testes and flatulence.
• Kapha, like the moon, influences an ebb and flow of body tides, body fluids, brain secretions.
• Pitta is related to the liver, bile, spleen, heart and eyes.

As with all things, our constitutions change over time. It is believed that imbalances in the doshas create many of our physical and mental illnesses, and that all disease begins with an imbalance or stress in the consciousness. Ayurvedic insight encourages a progressive approach to total well-being, where adjustments to lifestyle can create holistic balance. Ayurveda emphasizes a mind-body-spirit integration, seeking to treat the "whole" person, not a symptom. One should maintain a nurturing balance among the tri-dosha through diet and herbal remedies, in addition to aromas, yoga, meditation, sleep and pranayama. Bring metaphysical aspects of healing in your practice, such as the power of intention and the belief that we naturally gravitate toward wellness.

The simplicity of this approach influences the consciousness itself. Ayurvedic wisdom teaches that the qualities of nature fall within three groups – sattva, rajas and tamas – and that everything is made up of these groups in differing degrees. We are what we eat; we are what we think. Food nourishes both the body and the mind. This preventative way of living is being embraced by more and more people as science confirms we can enhance health and, in some cases, prevent problems through this down-to-earth wisdom of self-discipline, patience and commitment.

• Devote time to sleep, and ease into the day with meditation.
• Have a steady yoga practice, develop your sadhana.
• Clean more than teeth – floss, brush gums and scrape the tongue.
• Fill half the stomach. The right diet is healing therapy, the Ayurveda way.
• Eat fresh foods peacefully, either raw or with little cooking (raw for a short time to detox).
• Raw foods increases vata (air), cooked foods increases kapha and pitta (earth, water, fire).
• Live in harmony with nature; as one advances spiritually, the desire for food lessens.
• Be positive, you must be aware of love and purpose in all your intentions and actions.

YOUR DOSHA SELF-ASSESSMENT

Determining Your Dosha, Your Constitution

Mark yourself on a scale between 1-7 for each question as follows –
<u>1-2 Doesn't really apply to you.</u>   <u>3-5 Sometimes applies to you.</u>   <u>6-7 Mostly applies to you.</u>

Tally your score for each of the three doshas. This will indicate which body type you mostly belong to. If one dosha is significantly higher than the others, you can consider yourself a single dosha type (e.g. vata 100, pitta 40, kapha 35). If no dosha is dominant, then you are likely a two-dosha type (e.g. vata 90, pitta 80, kapha 40). In rare instances, you might score similarly for all three. This makes you a three-dosha type, which is considered highly unusual. This assessment is an abbreviated version based on a similar questionnaire devised by the Maharishi AyurVeda Association of America. For a deeper understanding of the Ayurvedic system, it is recommended that you consult a practitioner of this Association.

Vata | Air & Ether

___ Do things quickly
___ Have a poor retentive memory
___ Am enthusiastic
___ Don't gain weight quickly
___ Quick learner
___ Have a fast, light walking style
___ Difficulty making decisions
___ Suffer from wind – constipation
___ Often have cold extremities
___ Frequently anxious and worried
___ Don't like cold weather
___ Talkative with fast delivery
___ Moody and emotional
___ Difficulty falling asleep
___ Dry skin especially in winter
___ Imaginative mind
___ Energetic in bursts
___ Easily excitable
___ Irregular habits
___ Learn quickly-forget quickly
___ Restless sleep
___ Eat on spur of moment
___ Restless inner feelings
___ Always doing something

Total vata score max 24x7=168

Kapha | Earth & Water

___ Mostly relaxed
___ People think me slow
___ Gain weight quickly, lose slowly
___ Reasonably calm and placid
___ Asthmatic, and sinus congestion
___ Need plenty of sleep
___ Sleep very deeply
___ Do not anger easily
___ Slow to learn but remember well
___ Tendency to put on weight
___ Cool and damp climate unsettling
___ Hair is dark, thick and wavy
___ Smooth, soft, light-colored skin
___ Large, heavy and solid body
___ Affectionate and forgiving
___ Feel heavy and tired after eating
___ Can endure physical hardship
___ Slow in walking style
___ Oversleep and slow to awaken
___ Slow and methodical in action
___ Slow eater, slow digestion
___ Others consider me sweet-natured
___ Excess mucus and phlegm
___ Not easily ruffled

Total kapha score max 24x7=168

Pitta | Fire & Water

___ Am efficient
___ Precise in actions
___ Favor an ordered life
___ Hot weather is often distressing
___ Perspire easily
___ Easily irritated
___ Hair is early graying or balding
___ Become angry quickly
___ Good appetite
___ Like regular meals
___ Considered stubborn or rigid
___ Regular bowel movements
___ Perfectionist in details
___ Easily impatient
___ Enjoy ice-cold drinks & ice creams
___ Feel too hot in warm rooms
___ Like challenges
___ Over-critical of myself – others
___ Persistent in things I want
___ Poor tolerance of others' opinions
___ Don't like spicy, hot foods
___ Easily angered
___ Have thin blonde/sandy/red hair
___ Become tired in hot weather

Total pitta score max 24x7=168

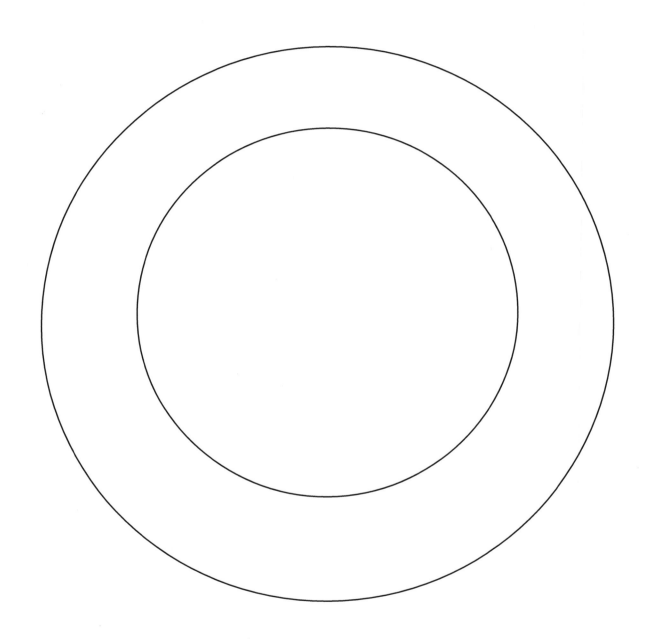

Vata – Air & Ether

Physical Characteristics

Lean and bony, protruding joints, lacking muscle, difficulty gaining weight, flexible, typically tall or short (not average height), dry skin, wrinkles with age, dry and brittle hair, long neck, thin red lips, narrow nose, lean hands (often cold), rough and weak nails, small eyes (typically dark), small mouths with large teeth (often crooked), dry and pale tongue.

Prone to arthritis, high or low blood pressure, cracking or popping joints, bladder/urinary disorders, muscle stiffness, headaches, insomnia, erratic eating, drinking, and sleeping habits, constipation, dizziness, ringing in ears, gas and bloating, premature aging, improper nutrient assimilation, poor stamina, attracted to vigorous exercise, strong interest in sex but quickly satisfied, impulsive behavior, chronic fatigue, heart disease, low energy, low back pain, intolerance of coldness and dryness, hoarseness of voice, food allergies, especially to wheat and dairy.

Mental Characteristics Balanced

Creative, artistic, compassionate, strong communicators, adaptable, emotionally sensitive, charismatic, perceptive, spontaneous, varied interests and abilities.

Mental Characteristics Unbalanced

Restless, forgetful, hyperactive, anxious, fearful, disorganized, prone to procrastination, moody and emotionally volatile, impatient, addictive personality.

Balancing

Keep warm, adhere to a vata diet, keep to a regular routine, get adequate rest (take naps and go to bed early), spend time in nature, meditate daily, avoid excess stimulation, follow creative and artistic passions, incorporate warming colors into your surroundings, listen to calming music.

Eating for Your Dosha

Seek out foods that are sweet, sour and salty. Sit down to eat and avoid eating on the run. Don't eat when nervous or anxious. Eat three or four smaller meals each day.

Eat a balanced breakfast with warm foods, warming spices, heavy whole grains (rice, wheat, quinoa), fresh fruit, heavy vegetables (squash, avocado) – cooked or steamed, fish, red meat (in moderation), nuts, water, fruit juices, herbal teas.

Avoid bitter, pungent and astringent foods, white sugar, caffeine, cold and carbonated beverages, light grains (corn, rye, puffed cereals), dry fruits (cranberries), gas inducing vegetables (broccoli, cauliflower, raw onion), beer and hard alcohol.

How to Heal the Body-Mind

Spend time in nature – swim, walk, golf, sail and bike. Nurture the body. Have an intention in your yoga practice and slow it down. Focus on strength and flexibility. Strengthen your Savasana practice.

Kapha – Earth & Water

Physical Characteristics
Broad frames, heavy bones, strong, shorter or taller than average, often overweight, smooth and oily skin, thick hair (often dark and curly), thick and clammy hands, large nose, strong nails, large mouths with white teeth, gentle eyes, long eyelashes, moderate appetite, slow metabolism and digestion, capable of vigorous activity (though avoids physical exertion), steady desire for sex, deep sleeper.

Prone to obesity, diabetes, colds, fluid retention, sinus congestion, anorexia and bulimia, allergies, asthma, excessive sleeping, lymphatic disorders, low thyroid function, intolerance to the cold, and heat disease.

Mental Characteristics Balanced
Patient, tolerant, forgiving, gentle, unhurried, loyal, accepting of others, strong stamina and endurance, good listeners, strong long-term memory.

Mental Characteristics Unbalanced
Possessive, lethargic, overly passive, envious, unable to express emotion, depressed, apt to give up easily, complacent, easily taken advantage of, fearful of letting go.

Balancing
Keep warm and dry, adhere to a kapha diet, eat light, get plenty of sleep at night (don't nap during the day), incorporate bright and vivid colors into your surroundings, listen to lively music, vary your daily routine, alternate cold showers with dry saunas, get plenty of vigorous exercise.

Eating for Your Dosha
Seek out foods that are bitter, pungent and astringent. Eat less in quantity and in frequency, eat at regular times each day.

Eat a light breakfast and a light evening meal, light, dry grains (toasted rye), warming spices, warm beverages, light fruits (pears, apples and dried fruits), vegetables (especially greens – broccoli, kale, eggplant), hot, spicy drinks (ginger or chai teas).

Avoid sweet, sour and salty foods, frequent snacking and late-night eating, white sugar, greasy foods, grains such as wheat, oats and rice, sour, juicy or heavy fruits (pineapple, oranges, and bananas), nuts (especially coconut, almonds, peanuts and walnuts), dairy, sweeteners, red meat.

How to Heal the Body-Mind
Exercise hard and often – speed walk, run, row, do martial arts, hike. Practice stimulating, intense, energizing yoga. Incorporate repetition into your daily routine and make sure to break a sweat. Work on opening the chest. Demand more from yourself. Resist the urge to rest during the day and during workouts. Don't put off achievements due to passivity. Concentrate intently in Savasana so you do not fall asleep.

Pitta – Fire & Water

Physical Characteristics
Medium build, average height and weight, developed and proportional muscles, little problem gaining or losing weight, oily skin, good stamina, fast metabolism and strong digestion, light-colored hair and eyes, soft nails, medium-sized hands, pointed nose, yellow teeth (prone to decay), often warm to the touch, determined stride, attracted to vigorous exercise and competitive sports, strong sexual appetite, easily aroused, light sleeper, low tolerance for hot weather or sunlight.

Prone to heavy perspiration, skin problems (such as acne, rashes, moles and freckles), hot and sweaty palms, excess hunger and thirst, canker sores, bleeding gums, sunburns, hot flashes, heartburn, inflammation, sore throats and tonsillitis, bad breath, appendicitis, bloodshot eyes, hepatitis, food allergies (especially nuts).

Mental Characteristics Balanced
Intelligent, confident, logically minded, courageous, funny, ambitious, joyful, articulate, skilled leaders, organized.

Mental Characteristics Unbalanced
Arrogant, manipulative, impatient, irritable, domineering, materialistic, perfectionistic, demeaning, overly competitive, judgmental.

Balancing
Keep cool, adhere to a pitta diet, meditate, do non-competitive and calming exercises (yoga, swimming, Tai Chi), listen to calming music, incorporate cooling colors into your surroundings, make time to rest daily, learn to appreciate others (do volunteer work), take cool showers, get in touch with your emotions, laugh often.

Eating for Your Dosha
Seek out foods that are sweet, bitter and astringent. Eat at regular times each day. Eat in a pleasing and calming environment. Drinking cool beverages and snacking on fresh vegetables regularly will help regulate body temperature.

Eat a balanced breakfast and an early lunch – grains, sweet, cooling and astringent fruits (pears, mango, apples), bitter and cooling vegetables (kale, broccoli, cucumber), milk, unsalted cheeses, water, herbal teas.

Avoid salty, sour and pungent foods, hot spicy food, refined sugar, alcohol, caffeine, sour fruits (grapefruit, pineapple), sour vegetables (mustard greens, tomatoes, radishes), nuts (especially peanuts, cashews, pistachios and all salted nuts), sour cream, red meat, shellfish, wine, hard alcohol, conducting business while eating.

How to Heal the Body-Mind
Get in a meditative state of mind – relax. Swim, walk, golf, sail, bike, ski. Choose a yoga that will help you surrender and relax. Work on cooling postures and seated twists. Strengthen your Savasana practice.

YOU, YOGA, AND FOOD
YOU BECOME WHAT YOU EAT AND HOW YOU LIVE

Our bodies are vessels for our Souls on this plane of existence. That being said, it's only logical that we keep these vessels in good health so they may sustain us on our path of developing ourselves to our highest potential. The food we eat plays a large part in maintaining the condition and wellness of our bodies, so it's of the utmost importance to pay attention to what we eat and why we eat it.

To say there is a single way in which to eat to bring about good health and wellness would be foolish. Just look at yoga itself. Within its practice, there are countless poses. A specific pose may or may not be suitable for every individual and the same can be said about food. Some foods may make us feel sluggish, while others may make us feel blocked. It is essential that we allow our bodies to tell us what to eat rather than consenting to diet rules told to us by someone else. Always keep in mind that food should supply us with both energy and clarity. A healthy diet will vary from person to person, but the effects should remain the same. We should feel healthy. We should sleep well. Our digestion should function properly. Our bodies and minds should feel supported rather than tapped by our yoga practice. It is all about conscious eating.

Once we understand that we should eat consciously, an intuitive sense of what is right and wrong in regard to our diet will surface. We can learn to recognize the foods our bodies need and when they need them. It's all about balance. There's a balance that can be found in what we choose to put in our bodies. Foods that feel good to our systems as we eat them, as well as after we've finished, are the foods we ought to eat. If we find ourselves experiencing an imbalance in our bodies, this is the perfect time to look back at what we've eaten that day or the day before and adjust our food intake until this sensation is alleviated.

Put aside for a second all the myths and theories you've heard about how you approach food within the practice of yoga and look at where they come from. A number of the ideas we've heard for years in the yoga community actually stem from either yogic scriptures or Ayurvedic beliefs. And if you don't know already, the concept of varying body types, each having their own necessary foods to flourish in the world, is a fundamental principle in Ayurveda. But many times the notion that few people are strictly one type is ignored or forgotten. So to apply a rigid idea of what a kapha type would benefit from to a person who is a mixture of that and vata type would be a disservice to that individual. We must therefore find, and this goes back to what is written above, a personal balance of foods to fit our own individual constitution.

We each possess an inherent wisdom that can guide us to a healthy diet. We simply need to listen as it will always tell us the truth. Eating should be about absorption, assimilation and elimination. Nothing more, nothing less. Eat when you feel hungry, don't when you don't. The foods we eat should be pure, wholesome and nutritious. To the yogi, food intake is for energy. Energy for fuel and energy for repair. A natural diet provides the best fuel for the body's functioning.

The Sun – All life on our planet receives its energy from the sun. It nourishes the plants that are eaten by the animals that are eaten by other animals. When we eat closer to the bottom of the food chain – fruits, vegetables, seeds, nuts, and grains, which are nourished directly from the sun, we receive a greater amount of the essential nutrients than by eating processed foods. Food derived directly from animals is almost a "second-hand" source of these nutrients, so make sure to eat plenty of items grown right from the earth. Also keep in mind that we, too, receive energy from the sun. Moderate sun exposure can provide us with a much needed dose of prana and vitamin D, which contributes to joint and bone health by helping the body absorb calcium. An hour per week should be more than enough to reap the benefits of the sun.

Plants – By the process of photosynthesis, plants use the sun's energy to combine water and carbon dioxide inside the chloroplasts, a plant's food factories, to make sugar. This process also produces oxygen as a byproduct.

Herbivores – Animals that eat a diet consisting of plants possess a long and complex digestive system with intestines 10 to 12 times the length of their body. Plants decay slowly and take a long time to digest so an internal system equipped for this is needed.

Carnivores – Animals with a diet consisting of meat have a simple and short digestive system with intestines a mere three times the length of the body. Since flesh decays very rapidly, the effects of which would poison the bloodstream, meat-eaters must have a system that swiftly expulses their food.

Fiber – Fiber is important for a healthy diet, digestive system and cholesterol levels. Foods containing fiber often have an abundance of other essential nutrients. Fruits, vegetables, legumes and whole-grain products are a good source of both soluble and insoluble dietary fiber.

Fruits and Vegetables – Eating your fruits and vegetables is one of the easiest ways to achieve a healthy diet. When our diets are rich with these types of foods, we can reduce the risk of heart disease and stroke, control our blood pressure and cholesterol, and guard against a number of ailments.

Carbohydrates – Our bodies need energy and the first place it will go is the carbohydrates we eat, the best of which are the complex carbohydrates, as they are stocked with vitamins and minerals. Carbohydrates do not only fuel the body, but also the mind. What do you think happens to the body and the mind when we restrict carbs?

Proteins – Protein is an important part of each cell in the body. It makes up your hair and nails. It's used to build and repair both muscles and tissues. It's a vital component of enzymes, hormones and other chemicals in the body. It's an essential building block of our bones, muscles, cartilage, skin and blood.

Fats – Not all fats are bad for you. Actually, we need a certain amount of fat in our diet. Monounsaturated fat is believed to lower cholesterol and may assist in reducing heart disease. Like polyunsaturated fat, it provides essential fatty acids for healthy skin and the development of body cells.

Dairy – Dairy is yet another important part of an individual's diet. An increase in dairy consumption can result in increased bone density, reduce the risk of osteoporosis, promote weight loss, lower blood pressure and help reduce the risk of hypertension.

EATING AND THE MIND

THE MORE YOU EAT, THE LESS FLAVOR; THE LESS YOU EAT, THE MORE FLAVOR. ~ CHINESE PROVERB

Now that we've come to understand that yoga is a balancing act of the mind, how can we restore that balance through the implementation of a healthy diet? While yoga focuses primarily on the mind, Ayurvedic teaching would have us direct our attention on maintaining balance through the functions of our bodies, as applied to the three doshas. The body cannot function properly if the mind is cloudy or over-active; thus one cannot perform optimally without the other. In order to reap the greatest benefits of yoga or Ayurvedic principles, we must understand how the two practices are connected. In other words, eat good, feel well.

Ayurvedic eating offers the foundation of the Six Tastes – sweet, sour, salty, bitter, pungent and astringent. It follows the simple philosophy of eating what naturally tastes appealing to us while avoiding that which contains harsh chemicals or toxins.

Each taste provides its own set of nutritional qualities. If you design your diet around the Six Tastes, you will incorporate all of the nutrients needed for sustainable health, growth and wellness.

How do we balance the doshas using the approach of the Six Tastes? Once we recognize the tastes that aggravate our dosha, we must work to decrease our intake of foods with such qualities. Simultaneously, we need to increase the consumption of tastes that provide balance.

Balancing Tastes	Vata	Pitta	Kapha
	Sweet	Sweet	Pungent
	Sour	Bitter	Bitter
	Salty	Astringent	Astringent

Aggravating Tastes	Vata	Pitta	Kapha
	Bitter	Sour	Sweet
	Pungent	Salty	Sour
	Astringent	Pungent	Salty

The primary intention of Ayurvedic nutrition is to incorporate each of the Six Tastes into every meal we eat. With a mindful awareness of the tastes that appeal to our doshas and the tastes we are less drawn to, we are able to strike the collective balance that our bodies and minds so deeply desire.

HOW THE GUNAS FEED US

WE KNOW WHAT WE ARE, BUT KNOW NOT WHAT WE MAY BE. ~ WILLIAM SHAKESPEARE

The three gunas – sattva, rajas and tamas – serve as the fundamental qualities (states) we float between throughout our lives. Together they balance and center us, but separately they lead us down very different paths. If we let ourselves become too tamasic, harboring sloth-like tendencies, we will lose not only our mental clarity but our physical health as well. A tamasic diet consists primarily of those foods that many would deem to be the most toxic for our bodies. However, if we let ourselves surrender to a primarily rajasic or overactive diet, we run the risk of becoming too restless and overstimulated. Perhaps it may help to think of this state as being too "caffeinated."

With sattva as our desired state, it must be said that we can only achieve it by eating solely that which will give us pure, positive energy. This is the reason why many yogis abide by a strict vegetarian diet and omit anything that may upset or aggravate the body.

Gunas Foods	Sattva	Rajas	Tamas
	Milk	Coffee, Black Tea	Red Meat
	Herbal Tea	Chicken	Alcohol
	Ghee	Eggs	Fast Food
	Grains	Onion, Garlic	Fried Food
	Fresh Sweet Fruits	Dark Lentils	Frozen Food
	Fresh Veggies	Citrus Fruits	Canned, Stale Food
	Honey	Very Spicy Foods	Refined Sugars
	Nuts	Chocolate	Tobacco
	Mung Beans	Salt	Soda

An array of attributes are associated with poor dietary choices. Fear, alienation and isolation are all examples of feelings one with an overly tamasic diet may experience. Similarly, one who is stuck in a rajasic state and a rajasic diet may experience feelings of impatience, stubbornness and power-seeking.

Different dietary tendencies also lead to varying behaviors. Tamasic eaters tend to overeat while rajasic eaters eat too quickly. Both have negative impacts on the body. The objective of sattva is to obtain peace while eating.

To achieve this state of peace, we must dedicate ourselves to a daily personal routine. This routine helps shift our bodies, minds and diets in the proper direction – meditation, spiritual practice, proper hygiene, walks in nature, control of senses, maintaining awareness to actions. In accordance with these practices, we begin to awaken ourselves to the contrasting, yet balancing roles of the gunas.

EAT THE SIX TASTES OF LIFE

WATER IS THE DRIVING FORCE OF ALL NATURE. ~ LEONARDO DA VINCI

Sweet Foods Build Tissues and Calm Nerves
Whole Grains
Starchy Vegetables
Dairy
Chicken, Fish
Honey, Molasses

Sour Foods Slow the Emptying of the Stomach, Regulating the Insulin Response
Citrus Fruits
Berries
Tomatoes
Pickled Foods
Vinegar

Salt Helps Stimulate Digestion
Table Salt
Soy Sauce
Salted Meats
Fish

Bitter Foods Loaded With Phytochemicals and Anti-inflammatories Help to Detoxify the Body
Green Leafy Vegetables
Kale
Celery
Broccoli
Sprouts
Beets

Pungent Foods are Anti-inflammatory and Stimulate Digestion and Metabolism
Peppers, Chillies
Onions, Garlic
Black Pepper
Cayenne, Curry, Turmeric
Cloves, Ginger, Mustard

Astringent Foods Absorb Water and Tighten our Tissues
Lentils
Beans
Green Apples
Grape Skins
Cauliflower
Pomegranates
Tea, Coffee

EAT THE COLORS OF THE RAINBOW

THERE IS NO PLACE LIKE HOME. ~ THE WONDERFUL WIZARD OF OZ

Red
Apple, Cherry, Cranberry
Guava, Nectarine, Persimmon
Papaya, Pink Grapefruit, Pomegranate
Raspberry, Red Grape, Strawberry
Watermelon, Beet, Radish
Red Cabbage, Red Pepper, Red Potato
Rhubarb, Tomato, Chili Pepper

Orange
Apricot, Cantaloupe, Mango
Orange, Tangerine, Carrot
Pumpkin, Sweet Potato, Yam

Yellow
Yellow Apple, Lemon, Mango
Papaya, Peach, Yellow Pear
Pineapple, Yellow Watermelon, Banana
Butternut Squash, Corn, Rutabaga
Yellow Pepper, Yellow Squash, Yellow Tomato

Green
Green Apple, Green Grape, Honeydew Melon
Kiwi, Lime, Artichoke
Asparagus, Avocado, Broccoli
Brussels Sprout, Cucumber, Celery
Arugula, Green Bean, Green Cabbage
Green Lettuce, Green Onion, Green Peas
Green Pepper, Kale, Spinach, Zucchini

Blue and Purple
Blackberry, Raspberry, Blueberry
Fig, Plum, Prune
Purple Grape, Raisin, Beet
Eggplant, Red Cabbage, Purple Cabbage

White
Pear, Coconut, Banana, Dates
White Nectarine, White Peach
Cauliflower, Potato, White Radish, Turnip
Parsnip, Onion, Garlic, Mushroom

SIX QUALITIES OF DOSHAS

FOR YOGA, INQUIRE WITHIN

Ayurvedic principles focus intently on the restoration of balance within the body. Given its direct connection between our bodies and the environment, food is one of the most important facets of that restoration.

In Ayurvedic teaching, the term "agni" (the literal translation is "fire") represents the release of energy that transpires inside our bodies through the processes of digestion, absorption and distribution. The term "fire" does not represent an actual flame, but rather the energy or heat that is responsible for bringing about a biological change within the body.

This positive or negative biological change is subject to the foods we eat. Although our diet may seem balanced, if we are not in tune with the state of our agni, we may be the culprit of our own imbalances. According to Ayurvedic teaching, the doshas contain six qualities associated with food – heavy and light, hot and cold, dry and oily.

Personal diets must be established based on the state of our agni in order to keep us healthy and, above all, balanced. Each dosha is equipped with its prescribed qualities. Though we desire to follow the guidelines of our dosha, it's important to keep in mind that not everyone fits one mold and certain people may harbor qualities of multiple doshas. The best way to restore and maintain balance is to know your dosha and be cognizant of your agni.

Heavy kapha	**Light** vata and pitta
Hot pitta	**Cold** vata and kapha
Dry vata	**Oily** pitta and kapha

Ayurveda characterizes physical illness as an imbalance. In effect, someone is extremely pitta or extremely kapha, that is to say, there is an increase in their dosha. To correct this imbalance we must increase or decrease the element in question. Ayurvedic teaching stresses that it is always easier to increase an element that is low through food intake than it is to decrease.

FOOD LOG

Eating healthy and balanced is easy in yoga training. But what about when you return home? Here is your next step after training. Keep a week-long food diary and reflect on what your diet looks like in the real world where imbalances might persist.

Example – Sunday

Meal #1 _____ Time of the day _____ What You Ate _____
Would you say this meal was more: Heavy ____ Light ____ Hot ____ Cold ____ Dry ____ Oily ____
Would you say this meal was more: Sattva ____ Rajas ____ Tamas ____
I choose this food because: It was nutrient dense ____ I had a craving ____

Meal #2 _____ Time of the day _____ What You Ate _____
Would you say this meal was more: Heavy ____ Light ____ Hot ____ Cold ____ Dry ____ Oily ____
Would you say this meal was more: Sattva ____ Rajas ____ Tamas ____
I choose this food because: It was nutrient dense ____ I had a craving ____

Meal #3 _____ Time of the day _____ What You Ate _____
Would you say this meal was more: Heavy ____ Light ____ Hot ____ Cold ____ Dry ____ Oily ____
Would you say this meal was more: Sattva ____ Rajas ____ Tamas ____
I choose this food because: It was nutrient dense ____ I had a craving ____

Meal #4 _____ Time of the day _____ What You Ate _____
Would you say this meal was more: Heavy ____ Light ____ Hot ____ Cold ____ Dry ____ Oily ____
Would you say this meal was more: Sattva ____ Rajas ____ Tamas ____
I choose this food because: It was nutrient dense ____ I had a craving ____

Meal #5 _____ Time of the day _____ What You Ate _____
Would you say this meal was more: Heavy ____ Light ____ Hot ____ Cold ____ Dry ____ Oily ____
Would you say this meal was more: Sattva ____ Rajas ____ Tamas ____
I choose this food because: It was nutrient dense ____ I had a craving ____

Food Group – fill in one cirle for each serving you ate.

Water   ○○○○○○○○○○○○
Green Vegetables ○○○○○○○○○○○○
Vegetables   ○○○○○○○○○○○○
Fruits   ○○○○○○○○○○○○
Beans & Legumes ○○○○○○○○○○○○
Meat   ○○○○○○○○○○○○
Dairy   ○○○○○○○○○○○○
Nuts & Seeds   ○○○○○○○○○○○○
Grains   ○○○○○○○○○○○○
Fats   ○○○○○○○○○○○○
Junk Foods   ○○○○○○○○○○○○

Yoga's History and Methods

To truly understand a complex subject like yoga, it's important for yoga teachers to study its roots. History provides context, such as how yoga influenced some of the great religions of the world. In our modern society, we can practice asanas, but lack understanding of the deeper context of how yoga applies to our personal journey through this lifetime.

Although the exact origins of yoga are unknown, it is thought to be about 5,000 years old. The earliest signs of the practice can be traced to what is now known as Pakistan, where stone sculptures were discovered of figures in traditional poses and meditation. The earliest traces of written reference to yoga came about 3,500 years ago in the form of the Vedas. The Vedas are texts about yoga, sacrifice and rituals, and were important in the formation of early Indian civilization. Later, the Vedic period gave way to the age of the Upanishads, where ancient philosophers turned their attention inward. Here the roots of Hinduism, Buddhism and Jainism formed with commentary on the ultimate reality and path to liberation. This is the basis of yoga being a philosophy, a psychological method, in recognizing that our senses are designed to draw us outward. The goal of yoga is to instill quiet in the mind to, learn to draw our senses back inward, in order to reach ultimate realization.

Yoga is lineage-based. When we understand where we are from, we can discover where we are going. In this foundational training, we practice a variety of yoga lineages – not to be highly skilled and experienced, but to understand the energetics that each brings to the practitioner.

Overall the lineage is Hatha yoga for the training I lead. But remember the commentary in Ayurveda on the doshas? How does one work with an individual within a group setting to bring them what they need in a class? With knowledge of the various systems of yoga, one can help to balance the dosha of an individual, offering different levels of practice to build confidence and calm, balance and serenity to almost any individual who commits to the process.

Yoga is not one-size-fits-all. It is, however, inclusive of all ages, body types, cultures and religions, requiring the skill to teach to the individual. My approach to yoga is adaptable and attainable for all practitioners. Be it children's yoga, senior's yoga, chair yoga for those desk-bound or with less balance, restorative yoga or therapeutic yoga.

Any serious yoga teacher will want to further their studies in these specialties as they find their calling or the need for yoga with these populations in their areas. Kids want to have fun. Adults want to learn to slow down and relax. Seniors think about their spiritual lives while also wanting to keep their bodies healthy. When we have the understanding of the context of yoga, it provides a deep reservoir of language for use in setting intentions and guiding others, no matter who they are, through their physical practice.

YOGA'S HISTORY TO MODERN DAY

WE ARE ALL JUST WALKING EACH OTHER HOME ~ RAM DAS

A segment of the Upanishads reads, "When the five senses and the mind are still and reason itself rests in silence, then begins the path supreme." This calm steadiness of the senses is called yoga.

Hundreds of years passed and the Upanishads developed what is now known as the four schools of yoga. The first two schools are Karma yoga (the path of action of the Soul) and Jnana yoga (yoga of the mind), both of which teach that the Ego or Self must be sacrificed to attain liberation. Karma yoga is the path of selfless devotion and service. By performing actions without wanting reward or payment, the yogi tries to free himself from the seemingly endless wheel of births and deaths. Jnana yoga is the path of intellectual knowledge and wisdom. This philosophical approach demands the study of the Upanishads. The last two schools are Bhakti yoga and Raja yoga. Bhakti yoga, the path of unconditional love and devotion, includes chanting and prayer which sublimates the emotions and channels them into devotion. Raja yoga, the path of meditation or mental control, is also seen as the scientific or step-by-step approach, hence it is also referred to as Ashtanga yoga, meaning eight-limbed or eight-stepped.

Later came Tantra yoga, a radical departure from the four schools of yoga. Focusing on the devotional aspects of Bhakti yoga, Tantra yoga teaches the union of opposites, showing the ultimate union as that of the Shakti female energy and the Shiva male energy. The emphasis is on the channeling of energy within to discover the evolution of the Self. Hatha, which branched out from Tantra, was interested in the transformation and union of the physical and subtle bodies to attain enlightenment. The very word Hatha is made up from the Sanskrit syllables "ha" for sun and "tha" for moon. It was also at this time that Patanjali, the father of modern yoga, wrote his famous "Sutras," which explain how we transform ourselves through yoga practice by following the eight steps or eight limbs. Patanjali also believed in Kriya yoga, the art of internally changing into a higher form.

All yoga styles teach contorting, stretching, bending, flexing and deep breathing at the same time. This practice has been around for more than 5,000 years and was originally developed from the Hindu philosophy. The word yoga comes from the work yoke and means "to bind" or "union." Originally, yoga was meant to "find the union of the individual with the divine means." This can be accomplished with the yoga lifestyle – proper diet, exercise, breathing, posture and meditation. There are many reasons why yoga has become so popular. Physically, yoga creates long, lean muscles and promotes serious flexibility. Mentally, yoga works wonders on stress. Spiritually, yoga centers you and bring you closer to the divine. The right style and teacher are different for various people. Studying all styles is recommended to give you an overview of the complete yoga offering of today. Yoga is wonderful for building up the immune system, overall physical health and mental stamina, naturally calming and healing the body, mind and Soul.

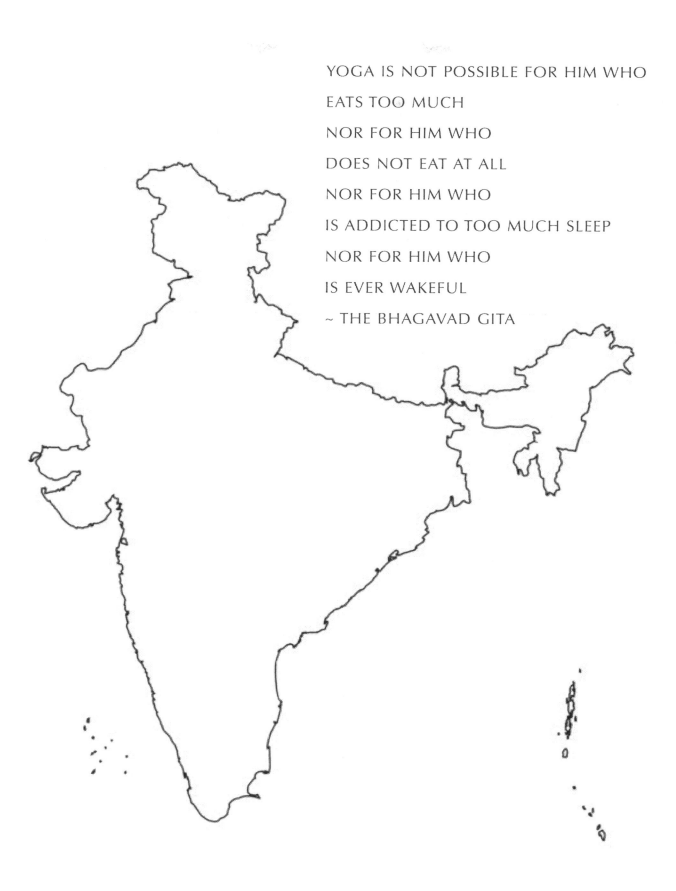

YOGA IS NOT POSSIBLE FOR HIM WHO

EATS TOO MUCH

NOR FOR HIM WHO

DOES NOT EAT AT ALL

NOR FOR HIM WHO

IS ADDICTED TO TOO MUCH SLEEP

NOR FOR HIM WHO

IS EVER WAKEFUL

~ THE BHAGAVAD GITA

The Four Main Older Styles of Yoga

Bhakti yoga is the path of devotion, by constant love, thought and service of the Divine. Bhakti yoga can be practiced by everyone. All that is needed is faith and constant remembrance of God.

Karma yoga is to be fully connected to life in service to others; the path of action and selfless service. Serving without attachment to the results of the action.

Jnana yoga is the yoga of wisdom. Through the knowledge of what really exists, that is, what is not changeable, one realizes Oneness with the entire Universe.

Raja yoga is balance and control of the mind through ethical practices, concentration and meditation.

The Newer Styles Created To Blend With Society

Tantra yoga draws from yoga science to unlock the practitioner's potential so that the light of knowledge is revealed and they may achieve their best life possible.

Kundalini yoga is fundamental to Tantra. It is the only form of yoga that requires a guru.

Hatha yoga focuses on the physical body. Seeing the body as a temple to be kept clean for health, healing and spiritual enlightenment. Asanas are for flexibility, pranayama for transformation and meditation to develop a mental compass.

Modern Yoga as We Know it Today

1893 – Swami Vivekananda at a World Parliament of Religion meeting at the Chicago World's Fair introduced "Raja yoga." In 1894, Swami Vivekananda started Vedanta classes in New York. The dominant Hindu monastic philosophy was rooted in ancient Vedic teachings. In 1899, Swami Vivekananda founded the Vedanta Society in New York. Postures known as "Hatha yoga" were given little attention as they were considered the least important component of yoga practice.

1920s – T. Krishnamacharya (1888-1989) began his studies with the Yoga Sutras. Because so little was known about yoga postures, his journey led him to Tibet to find a guru to study with. At some point his father began to guide him along this path, but the exact origins of his practice are unknown. One thing we all agree on is that Krishnamacharya became the Father of modern-day Hatha yoga, a famous yogi and philosopher of the twentieth century who taught his son, T.K.V. Desikachar, as well as Indra Devi, Pattabhi Jois and B.K.S. Iyengar.

1920s – Paramhansa Yogananda (1893-1952) was the first yoga master to take up permanent residence in the West. Arriving in America in 1920, he traveled throughout the United States on his campaign teaching the value of balancing the material with the inner, spiritual life. His lasting impact is his "Autobiography of a Yogi." He founded the Self-Realization Fellowship in 1946 as well as Kriya yoga, the path of Karma, Jnana and Bhakti yoga.

1940s – Iyengar yoga was developed in the 1940s in India by B.K.S. Iyengar. Iyengar yoga is known as the yoga for alignment of the body. Standing poses are very important to strengthen and align the body. Holding poses is important to experience the pose. Teachers use props to accommodate each pose for each student. Iyengar is known for its focus on proper skeletal alignment and attention to detail. Props such as belts, blocks and blankets help you deepen a pose while emphasizing precision allowing one to increase flexibility over time. This is a great yoga discipline to practice along with physical therapy because it focuses on the movements of the joints. Poses are sometimes held for a minute or more to work on skeletal and muscular alignment.

1947 – Developed by Pattabhi Jois in 1947, Ashtanga yoga is comprised of six progressively difficult series of poses. Ujjayi breathing is very important, aiding in internal cleansing. Rooms are heated to over 90 degrees, sweating helps to detox the body, the internal body heat helps to thin the blood creating better circulation, and heated thinned blood helps to lubricate joints and cleans internal organs. Pattabhi Jois "Guruji" was born in Mysore, India, in 1915. Pattabhi Jois said yoga is 99% practice and 1% theory. He studied under Krishnamacharya, who discovered the 2,000-year-old texts of Ashtanga yoga written on palm leaves.

1959 – Sivananda yoga is one of the largest schools of yoga in the world. Sivananda yoga calls for the rigorous application of the five points of yoga – proper exercise, breathing exercises, relaxation, vegetarian diet and the study of scriptures/meditation. Sivananda yoga promotes the teachings of the ancient science of yoga, both mind and body, as a positive guide to improve health, happiness and spiritual well-being.

1966 – Kripalu yoga, the yoga of consciousness, was developed by Swami Kripalu, who studied Kundalini yoga in India. In the 1960s, Swami Kripalu brought his yoga to America, establishing the first Ashram, Yogaville, in Pennsylvania. Students learn to focus on the mental and physical reaction to the various poses. They develop on three stages – learning the pose, holding the pose and the combination of the pose into a meditation in motion.

1966 – Integral yoga, Sri Swami Satchidananda Ashram, Yogaville

1968 – Yogi Bhajan introduced his own brand of Kundalini yoga into the United States.

1970s – Bikram yoga, Yin yoga

1983 – T.K.V. Desikachar, son of Krishnamacharya, resisted the yoga world and finished college with a degree in engineering. After college, his eyes were opened to the benefits of yoga and he studied with his father and developed what he called Viniyoga. It was yoga tailored to fit the needs of the individual and joins breath with movement. Flowing with inhalations and exhalations, this yoga is somewhere between B.K.S. Iyengar's precision and Pattabhi Jois' Ashtanga workout.

1980s – Forrest yoga, Jivamukti yoga, Baptiste yoga

1997 – Ansura yoga

TIBETAN YOGA
THE FORGOTTEN YOGA

Marianne's Updated Five Tibetans

Tibetan One
• Stand in mountain with out stretched arms, circles of the arms 1 – 21x
• Rest in Mountain for several breaths

Tibetan Two
• On back, feet flexed over hips and arms at side spalms down, lift legs and head 1 – 21x
• Rest in Shavasana for several breaths

Tibetan Three
• Kneel, balls feet ground, hands at buttocks, chin tucked and exhale, inhale to open throat 1 – 21x
• Rest in child's pose for several breaths

Tibetan Four
• Sit in staff with chin tucked and inhale, exhale to reversed table 1 – 21x
• Rest in forward fold for several breaths

Tibetan Five
• Up dog with toes tucked and inhale, exhale to down dog 1 – 21x
• Rest on belly for several breaths

Traditional Tibetan Prayer
May I be at peace.
May my heart remain open.
May I know the beauty of my own true nature.
May I be healed.
May I be a source of healing in this world.

TANTRA YOGA
AUSPICIOUS CONSCIOUSNESS SUPREME BLISS

The Tantra yoga tradition had been one of the potent powers for spiritual enlightenment of the Hindus for thousands of years. All persons without the distinctions of caste, creed or color may draw inspiration and attain spiritual strength, wisdom and eternal bliss.

Tantra yoga focuses on devotion and worship of the Goddess. Tantric yogis believe that human suffering comes from the illusion of opposites and from the mistaken notion that the Self is somehow separate from the objects it desires. Tantrics see all possible sets of opposites, good and evil, hot and cold, hard and soft, male and female, and that it is these opposites that are contained within the universal consciousness.

Tantric yogis believe that the only way a yogi can liberate himself from suffering is to unite the opposites in his own body. They believe that the physical body is a sacred temple to the Divine, a vehicle for attaining liberation. Ultimate unity, final liberation or samadhi, is the internal merging of the male energy of Shiva with the female principle Shakti. Maybe the nicest part of the Tantric way of living is the belief that the female energy makes liberation possible.

The Practice
- Asana – Emphasis on the development of the powers latent in the first six chakras.
- Pranayama – Designed to channel Divine energy.
- Bandhas – Used to awaken Shakti energy.
- Mudras – There are 108 total mudras in Tantra yoga.
- Visualization – Especially of one's deity present for the purpose of expanded awareness.
- Mantra – Transforming us to freedom.
- Yantra or Mandala – Contains a seed center, which represents the union of the cosmos and the mind, concentric circles, which represents the various levels of existence, and a square fence with four gates to protect the sacred space.

KUNDALINI YOGA

MAY THE LONG TIME SUN SHINE UPONE YOU, ALL LOVE SURROUND YOU, AND THE PURE LIGHT WITHIN YOU, GUIDE YOUR WAY HOME ~ SAT NAM

The practice of Kundalini yoga is said to have been created over 50,000 years ago in India and Tibet by a group of rishis, or Vedic sages, who found through a series of postures, movements, breathing and verbal techniques that a person could access and utilize their own personal power.

Kundalini refers to the potential psychic energy, Kundalini energy, that dwells dormant in our bodies. It is said to reside at the base of our spine, coiled like a serpent in our first chakra, waiting to be awakened. Through the practice of Kundalini yoga, this energy is stimulated to move upwards through the six other chakras. As it climbs from one chakra to the next, the practitioner also ascends from one rung to the next up the yogic ladder. The higher the Kundalini energy travels, the further the practitioner advances spiritually. When this energy reaches the seventh chakra, there occurs a unification of the divine energy and the cosmic Self.

In 1969, these sacred teachings were brought to the West by Yogi Bhajan, founder of 3HO (Happy, Healthy, Holy Organization). It was the first time that Kundalini yoga was not only taught publicly, but also written down and offered to anyone wanting to practice. It had been maintained as a secret oral tradition for thousands of years which gave it an air of mystery. Customarily, those seeking to learn would serve a master and prove their devotion before becoming a true student. It took time and patience, but the rewards were said to be great.

Most of the practitioners of Kundalini yoga believe it to be the most powerful and inclusive of the twenty-two schools of yoga. It is said to give up to 16 times faster results than that of Hatha yoga as it does not rely on such difficult poses. The practice consists of a sequence of asanas that have been combined with pranayama, mudras, bhandas, meditation and mantras. As an example, the mantra "Ong Namo Guru Dev Namo" is chanted at least three times before beginning any practice and the mantra of "sa ta na ma" is chanted throughout class to the beat of body movements.

Commonly, Kundalini yoga teachers advise to practice only under the supervision of a knowledgeable and qualified teacher. They believe that awakening Kundalini without guidance can bring about mental confusion, mood swings, egotism and psychosis, when a person is thought to have been "bitten by the snake."

As our society becomes increasingly technological, our world becomes more intimately connected and influenced by its numerous cultures. The pace of change is on the rise and the stress on our body's nervous system is increasing. The science of Kundalini yoga allows us to tap into a technology that helps us cope with this escalating change. The inner science of the mind is the tool that will enable us to cope with the pressure of these changes. It is the mind that interprets our outer and inner worlds, and it is the mind that we must train to guide us through the flow of change.

The Practice
• Kriyas and meditations designed to tune into Self-awareness
• Postures to awaken the spine
• Breath and bandha work to aid in the flow of energy

HATHA VINYASA FLOW YOGA
EVERYTHING HAS A BEGINNING, MIDDLE, END: THE MOMENT HAS A STOPPING POINT, THE BREATH DOES NOT

Where are We? Deepen Self-Awareness Through Repetition

Repetition of breath. Repetition in and out of postures. According to the Ashtanga tradition, the purpose of linking breath with movement is internal cleansing. Vinyasa generates the subtle internal heat of digestive fire. This transformational fire not only digests food but also creates experiences and sensations. The internal and external heat from this practice helps to remove impurities. The breath used in vinyasa, ujjayi, creates a vibration across the soft palate of the mouth, warming the breath as it enters the body. Muscles work in balance. On the way into a posture, we work the agonist muscles. On the way out of a posture, we work the antagonist muscles. Through breath, postures and repetition, our circulation increases.

Establish the Self in the Present Through Acceptance of the Form of the Posture Today

Most people think the word vinyasa means "flow," some think it means "steps," still others interpret the word as "vi" "in a special way" and "nyasa" "to place." With all these interpretations out there, you can see the importance of adapting the postures to the individual. We must understand the individual, where they have been, where they are present, and where they wish to go. Having said that, the most common understanding of vinyasa is the linking of body movement with breath, where breath and movement are seamlessly united in such a way that each beginning is formed from the previous ending.

Set a Direction for the Future With a Plan

"Take a vinyasa" is a common phrase used by teachers in class. Students have time to do what their bodies need in that particular practice. Moving through space, the rhythm of the spine breath initiates movement from a calm energy. Having said this, if you as the teacher create vinyasa plans, they must be tailored to fit each individual. For this, you must understand mindfully where the person has been, where they are currently, and where they wish to go.

Actualize Full Potential of Your Journey With Enlightenment

Practice. Practice. Practice. As my father has tailored his famous saying over the years, "Practice makes perfect, practice makes pretty darn good, just keep practicing, there is no such thing as perfect." Accept. Accept. Accept. Life is easier this way and you will always go with the flow!

Is Going Through Your Vinyasa Right for You?

_____

_____

_____

_____

_____

IYENGAR YOGA
EVERY POSE IS BOTH TADASANA AND SAVASANA ~ B.K.S. IYENGAR

B.K.S. Iyengar was my teacher.

Most people today attribute the use of yoga props to the work of Iyengar.

Technique
Iyengar has structured hundreds of classical asanas to enable beginners to progress safely – gaining flexibility, strength and awareness in body, mind and spirit.

Adjustments in the Alignment
Iyengar's dedication to correct alignment methods have influenced every style of yoga being practiced today. His methods provide a system to reduce the suffering of students, to enable the ability to gain awareness of how to feel in the asanas.

Sequence
Iyengar refined the therapeutic aspects of yoga asanas. He experimented on himself to cure his own weaknesses. The results were asana sequencing that has powerful cumulative effects on the practitioner. His method of holding postures so the benefits could penetrate deeper for the aid of the individual has influenced countless yoga teachers and practitioners worldwide.

Pranayma
Essential for true meditation, according to Iyengar, pranayma is needed to still the mind.
"The mind is the king of the senses, and the breath is the king of the mind."

Meditation in Action
Iyengar thought if one could meditate on a flame, why not a posture being practiced. In doing this, the mind becomes aware of different parts of the body, eventually becoming absorbed into the body as a whole.

Basic Yoga Props
• The Floor
• The Wall
• Chairs
• Tables
• Stair Case
• Balance Beam
• Blocks
• Straps
• Blankets
• Mats
• Bolsters
• Sandbags
• Rope Walls

ASHTANGA YOGA

ASHTANGA IS 99% PRACTICE AND 1% THEORY ~ PATTABHI JOIS

PHILOSOPHY WITHOUT PRACTICE IS NOT CONSIDERED TO BE TRUE PHILOSOPHY. ~ DAVID SWENSON

BEFORE YOU'VE PRACTICED THE THEORY IS USELESS. AFTER YOU'VE PRACTICED THE THEORY IS OBVIOUS. ~ DAVID WILLIAMS

The Ashtanga yoga method creates intense internal heat, which leads to profuse sweating that brings toxins from the body to the surface. Purifying the blood and stimulating circulation, the body is then purified from disease. After years of practice it is possible to purify the nervous system and the sensory organs and to gain increased mind awareness.

The Elements of The Ashtanga Practice

Ashtanga Opening Prayer
For the peaceful resolution of the deluding nature of repetitive existence,
I bow at the Gurus' lotus feet, and behold the awakened joy of my own Soul.
This is the ultimate refuge acting as a shaman for my spiritual enrichment.
OM shanti, shanti, shanti.

Tuning in With Breath
• Ujjayi pranayama

Focusing With Gazing Points
• Drishti – eyes, nose, navel, hand, thumb, toes, left, right, sky

Transforming Energy With Body Locks
• Bandhas – are used to seal energy in the body and make the practice light and strong.

The Six Series of Ashtanga Yoga
• Primary series – realigns and detoxifies, builds physical strength and a solid foundation.
• Intermediate series – strengthens the nervous system, purifies the nadis and chakras.
• There are four Advanced series' – that build Divine energy flow.

Ashtanga Closing Prayer
May all be well with mankind.
May all the leaders of the earth protect in every way by keeping to the right path.
May there be goodness for those that know the earth to be sacred.
May all the worlds be happy.
OM peace, peace, peace.

SALUTATIONS

HONOR THE SUN AND THE MOON AND UNIVERSAL LIFE ITSELF

The Sun Salutation

Traditionally practiced in the morning, the Sun Salutation is the most universal of all salutations. They are excellent because it stretches and strengthens all the major muscle groups in the body and exercises the respiratory system.

In Hindu mythology, the Sun God is worshiped as a symbol of health and immortality. The Sun Salutation gives reverence to the internal sun as well as to the external sun, the creative life force of the universe that the yogis believe to radiate inside as well as outside the body.

The Sun Salutation limbers up the whole body in preparation for the asanas. It is a graceful sequence of twelve positions linked by a continuous flowing motion and accompanied by five deep breaths. Each position counteracts the one before, stretching the body in a different way and alternately expanding and contracting the chest to regulate the breathing. One round of Sun Salutations consists of two sequences, the first leading with the right foot, the second leading with the left. Coordinate your movement with your breathing. Start by doing three rounds and gradually build up to twelve.

As always in yoga, do it slowly and consciously. Sun Salutation benefits are an established state of concentration and calm. Other benefits include – stretching of the abdominal and intestinal muscles, exercising the arms and spinal cord, aiding in the prevention and relief of stomach ailments, reducing abdominal fat, improving digestion and circulation, creating a more limber spine, toning the abdomen, and muscles of the legs, and strengthening of the nerves and muscles of the chest, shoulders, arms and legs.

The Sun Salutation

Step 1: Begin standing with hands in prayer position at the heart center
Step 2: Inhale, extend arms overhead
Step 3: Exhale, forward fold
Step 4: Inhale, step right foot back
Step 5: Retain breath, step left foot back into plank
Step 6: Exhale, lower body toward floor
Step 7: Inhale, into cobra or updog
Step 8: Exhale, downward dog
Step 9: Inhale, right foot forward
Step 10: Exhale, left foot forward
Step 11: Inhale, arms overhead
Step 12: Exhale, standing with hands in prayer position at the heart center

The Sun-Moon Salutation

The Sun-Moon Salutation is traditionally practiced at night on knees so the body is low to the floor.
This can be hard on some knees so pad them well. The Sun-Moon Salutation is excellent for beginners.

Step 1: Begin kneeling with hands in prayer position at the heart center
Step 2: Inhale, sun
Step 3: Exhale, table
Step 4: Inhale, cow
Step 5: Exhale, cat
Step 6: Inhale, cow
Step 7: Exhale, cat
Step 8: Inhale, down dog
Step 9: Exhale, extended child's pose
Step 10: Inhale, lift onto knees
Step 11: Exhale, prayer at heart center
Step 12: End kneeling with hands in prayer position at the heart center

The Moon Salutation

The lesser known of the salutations, the Moon Salutation, is easier on a tight body and traditionally
practiced at night. Because the moon holds female energy, this series is a balanced compliment to
the sun series. Again, twelve positions linked by a continuous flowing motion, moving with the breath.
One round of Moon Salutation consists of two sequences, the first leading with the left foot, the
second leading with the right. Start by doing three rounds and gradually build up to twelve.

Step 1: Inhale, standing star
Step 2: Exhale, bend to left
Step 3: Inhale, standing star
Step 4: Exhale, bend to right
Step 5: Inhale, standing star
Step 6: Exhale, goddess
Step 7: Inhale, straighten legs and arms out to side
Step 8: Exhale, easy side triangle to left
Step 9: Inhale, straighten legs and arms out to side
Step 10: Exhale, easy side triangle to right
Step 11: Inhale, straighten legs and arms out to side
Step 12: Exhale, hands in prayer position at heart center

PARTNER YOGA
BE OBLIGATED TO DO YOUR BEST, NOT OBLIGATED TO SUCCEED

Why Partner yoga? In order to truly understand practicing yoga with a partner, one must first ask why do it at all? Is it to get deeper into postures? To connect with another, perhaps with a special someone?

Partner yoga takes your practice to another level. Physically, emotionally, mentally and spiritually. It provides participants with the understanding that shared moments of connection and cooperation with a focus on breath, alignment and support lead to much more of the same over time.

Communication is the foundation to a strong partnership. Intimacy and touch is a basic human need. Discover a deeper connection with your partner through partner yoga.

But partner yoga isn't limited to couples. Having another person provide support with their body or added weight to the force of gravity allows one to move deeper into postures, to move past the feeling of straining to bend a little further. Let the weight of another allow your muscles to relax and extend certain postures that are limited due to tight muscles and joints. Much like sandbags are used as yoga props, consider a yoga partner as a human yoga prop, able to communicate with you and adjust to your individual needs.

The Experience
- Connect breath and body movement
- Warm up both bodies with partner flow
- Balance strength and flexibility
- Develop comfort and intimacy through shared breath, postures and eye contact
- Strengthen relationships – understand the power of communicating without words
- Surrender and effort are essential to bring balance
- Deepen your trust, security and sensitivity with one another
- Fun and laughter keeps the energy flowing
- Enjoy a fun, wholesome and supportive practice you can take off the mat
- Strength and conditioning – physical fitness
- Therapeutic Thai massage, come together with a purpose of opening up to learn and receive
- Savasana, Oneness is first finding the Divinity within, then sharing together

PRENATAL AND POSTNATAL YOGA
NEVER STAND WHEN YOU CAN SIT, NEVER SIT WHEN YOU CAN LAY DOWN, NEVER LAY DOWN WHEN YOU CAN TAKE A NAP

Prenatal yoga is a time to prepare and grow the most nuturing environment for both mother and baby. Pre and postnatal yoga should begin with caution at a low intensity, and always after receiving doctor's approval. The mother should never, ever, ever strain or push beyond her comfort limit. As the teacher, it is your job to pay very close attention as to how mom moves into and out of each posture. Remind both your pre and postnatal moms to drink lots of fluids all day long and always have them warm up and cool down gradually, at least five minutes at each end.

First Trimester is About Containment
The woman's body and yoga poses are all about containment, creating a space of strength and flexibility for the upcoming changes. Practice moving less deeply in each posture. I tell my students to try to move only 60% to 80% in each pose.

Second Trimester is About Nuturing
The woman's body and yoga poses are all about nature, creating a healthy natural environment for the baby. This is the time to begin avoiding putting pressure on major blood vessels and preventing oxygenated blood flow throughout the lower body. To accomplish this, we avoid prone (face down), supine (lying on your back), and any postures laying on the right side. Even Savasana is modified.

Third Trimester is About Expansion
The woman's body and yoga poses are all about expansion, allowing for safe expansion. Plenty of relaxation postures with breath awareness are advised. After week 34, no squatting poses. Now is the time to breathe health into mom and help her prepare for her upcoming job of giving birth.

Why Yoga is so Beneficial for Your Pregnancy
• Tones muscles and you teaches how to control them.
• Promotes understanding of breath control and what can be achieved by smooth rhythmic breathing.
• Teaches birthing techniques through mindful, rhythmic movement.
• Teaches self-taught relaxation.
• Emphasizes to never strain or push beyond one's comfort limit.
• Increases flexibility to the hip joints, necessary for giving birth.
• Teaches awareness and relaxation of muscles of the pelvic floor, encourages feeling of openness
• Tones and strengthens skeletal muscles, glands and organs of the body.

Things to Never do or to Avoid During in a Prenatal Yoga Practice
• If you have vein issues or blood clots, never do folded leg postures.
• Never lay on back or right side, modify Savasana and reclining postures especially later in pregnancy
• Avoid deep flexion or extension movements.
• Never hold your breath because this will limit oxygen to both mother and baby.
• Avoid heated environments that can raise your maternal core above 100.4 F.
• Avoid bouncy movements because of joint instability.

Postnatal Yoga is About Healing
After birth, postnatal yoga is all about helping mom recover. It is a time to use a mindful, moderate yoga practice to slowly bring strength and stability back into the body. Mom's body needs 6-8 weeks to begin any workout routine at all, so emphasize self-love and patience during this time.

YOGA FOR CHILDREN

THE MORE YOU DO FOR CHILDREN TODAY, THE LESS YOU WILL NEED TO DO FOR THEM TOMORROW

Birth to One Year
Parent and baby classes.

One to Five Years
Fun, Fun, Fun. Relate postures to the world around them.

Six to Ten Years
Still fun. Add in a little change for mental growth and physical development.

Middle School Years
Remember, this group is the "tweeners" – they think they are grown up, so make class groovy!

High School Years
Almost grown up, time to begin letting go.

Program Ideas
• Speak truths. Teach only what you feel deeply in your heart.
• Discuss real issues. Ask the children why they are in the class.
• Create a comfortable space. This is going to be a different experience for most.
• Yoga teaches us how to show respect. It begins with how we respect our own bodies' limits.
• Listen. Learn how to listen to ourselves and then how to listen to others.
• Self-image. Yoga will improve how you feel about yourself today.
• Yoga teaches how to accept one's own limits and that we all have a right to be here.
• Yoga teaches the value of self-esteem. How self-esteem is not fixed, it has peaks and valleys from posture to posture and day to day.
• Body image does not regulate the depth one can get into a posture. With the distorted view of body image today, yoga teaches that all bodies can move deeply into postures.
• Encourage children to become advocates for themselves. As they learn how to get into and out of postures, they learn how to resolve for themselves. The best part – they learn that self-reliance conquers any difficulty.
• Children have a lot of worries and pressures today. Teach them how to feel good and de-stress.
• Teach the reasons why we need to eat healthy, be active, get enough rest, relax and how to take care of ourselves.
• Above all, keep a sense of humor.
• If you want to teach in public schools, you will need to create a curriculum to present.

YOGA FOR SENIORS

AGE PUTS A LIMIT ON LIFE

I have a standing joke in my classes – if you are my age or younger, you have to do what I say.
If you're older, you have to try to do what I say. And if you are much older, you can do what you want.
And then I proudly tell my age.

For as long as I can remember, my goal in life was to be a wise old lady. I often kid that I'm in retirement, since my design for life was to teach yoga when I retired. In my mind, I always had this wonderful image of myself. It was of a white-haired lady sitting in a rocker on a moist, wooden porch with a smile of contentment with a life fully lived. So how do we go about teaching a person such as that? I believe the best way to even begin to answer this question is to understand the true reason why.

As we live longer and longer lives, the interest and need to lead an active, healthy life has grown exponentially. But one of the most predominant issues with this time of life is we tend to become more sedentary. This inactivity typically makes us more prone to a number of ailments which then lead us to even greater lengths of limited mobility. In turn, we become even more susceptible to these health issues and so the cycle begins.

Though we may have earned it, retirement isn't necessarily, in the strictest sense of the phrase, a "time to take life easy." When we adopt a sedentary lifestyle, our body takes the toll. Our muscles can shorten, our joints can weaken, and our circulation can worsen. We may experience osteoporosis due to a need for weight-bearing activities or a loss of balance due, in part, to long periods of sitting as opposed to standing. A remarkable tool to combat and improve these, among other, health issues is yoga.

Being yoga practitioners, we all know that many of our standard yoga postures can be extremely challenging for someone in their 20s, let alone for someone in their 70s. But with a few alterations, yoga can become a beneficial exercise of ease. It can be practiced in a chair or in a bed. Props like straps, blocks and pillows can aid a person into a pose and help them maintain a pose. The breath work can help get more oxygen to the brain, improving one's memory and learning capacity. It can reduce stress, relieve anxiety and improve disposition. Yoga can help emotionally, giving a person more control, confidence and a social outlet. The possibilities and benefits of yoga for our senior population are endless.

But how do we instill wisdom on a group in which we have not lived in? How do we give comfort to an age we have yet to experience? That is where your Soul comes into play.

RESTORATIVE YOGA
MENTAL HAPPINESS IS TOTAL RELAXATION

Restorative yoga is a traditional style of yoga that has been in use by practitioners of many styles for a long time. Iyengar spotlighted Restorative yoga and was instrumental in bringing it into the mainstream. In the 1960s, Yin yoga grew from Restorative yoga. These calmer styles of yoga are gaining in popularity because they work well for many people.

Restorative Postures Benefits
• Increases mobility in body – hips, spine, groin
• Increases flexibility in joints and connective tissue
• Releases fascia throughout the body
• Improves lubrication and protection of joints
• Aids digestion
• Relieves fatigue, soothes the nervous system, rejuvenates the body, refreshes the mind
• Helps with menstruation
• Reduces cardiac disorders
• Helps with TMJ and migraines
• Regulates energy in the body – helps to bring a restful state and restore energy
• Brings one into highest state of deep relaxation and consciousness
• Regulates the breath – calming and balancing to the mind and body
• Lowers stress levels
• Helps provide greater stamina
• Improves ability to sit for meditation
• Ultimately, you will have a better active practice

Restorative Postures Cautions
• Pregnant women should lay on their left side, and on an incline with their head above the abdomen when lying on their backs
• Students with heart conditions or high blood pressure must keep their hearts higher than their feet

Restorative Class Ideas

Introduction
- Postures are passive.
- Relax in each posture, soften muscles – fascia, focus is closer to the bones – a deeper access to the body
- Postures held for three to five minutes, even 20 minutes at a time.
- A more meditative approach to yoga that teaches you how to really listen to your body's signals while being very still.
- At times, you will be in an uncomfortable position. Restorative yoga asks you to learn to "be" and to "accept" in that given moment.
- This is an intimate and quiet practice – with reflection, stillness and focus on yourself. Feelings, sensations and emotions that can often be avoided or distract you in a fast-paced yoga practice will often arise in restorative yoga practice. Restorative yoga is often used in programs that deal with addictions, eating disorders, anxiety and deep pain or trauma.

Practice Principles
- Be the observer.
- Let go with gravity and universal life forces.
- Distinguish between pain and discomfort. What is pain? What is discomfort? Allow time, your breath and focus for the sensation to pass.

Asana Options
- Legs Up Wall – with or without props
- Dance – get blood moving
- Mountain – feel energy over body
- Forward Fold – blanket at hip flexors
- Corpse – with strap at knee and bolster under knees
- Reclining Big Toe Twist
- Reclining Alligator
- Reclining Bound Angle
- Reclining Hero
- Ball with eyes squinting into Bridge with eyes relaxed
- Bridge with block
- Hammock
- Supported Fish
- Easy Plow
- Easy Shoulder Stand
- Supported Pigeon
- Supported Frog
- Supported Child's Pose
- Table – dynamically in order to move the spine in six ways
- Deep Yin Twist – with bolster
- Sitting – dynamically in order to move the spine in six ways
- Sitting Wide Leg Forward Fold
- Sitting – inhale with hands at back of head, exhale with hands at heart center
- Sitting – gather energy at end of class
- Sitting – feel energy at end of class
- Lazy Dog – with lots and lots of props

Yoga Anatomy and Therapeutics

Really Real Yoga involves understanding the human body and beyond. Iyengar taught that we begin with the flesh and move toward the Soul. For most people, one's introduction to yoga begins with the physical body. In order to practice yoga and teach yoga safely, it is very important to understand our physical structure and function.

Understanding how we move and the implication for stress points along the kinetic chain are keys to being a successful and safe yoga instructor. Equally important is how to instruct others to move their bodies in space with clear and simple instruction. As one becomes ingrained in the study of yoga, they become students of life. This includes constantly seeking out many teaching concepts of applied yoga anatomy to bring into your practice and teaching. Good yoga teachers learn and share constantly.

Really Real Yoga doesn't need to name the poses in Sanskrit or even English. Moving and breathing speak a universal language. With a focus on the physics of movement, we emphasize the action of movement and the reaction of what occurs in the body. Breath is connected to movement, going beyond simply "inhale and exhale." If one is not connecting breath to movement, one is not practicing yoga. It's all about the breath.

I believe that the Soul resides in the space of our breath. It is important for us to connect mindfully with this space as we move through asana practice. Our breath is our teacher – our guide. Asana practice has stopping points – the breath never does – until our final one.

Proper focus on clear directions of movement – linked to breath – enables a yoga practitioner to move inward. Really Real Yoga is practiced without mirrors. It's hard to focus and reflect inward when you're distracted by the outward reflection of your hair, clothes and others. When you feel it, you simply know it. There's a difference between doing a pose and being in a pose. Real yoga strives for the latter.

Really Real Yoga focuses a lot of attention to the spine. The spine moves six ways and should be moved in every direction in each class. Given the spine's relationship to the diaphragm and lungs, emphasis is given in lengthening the spine, making space for the breath, allowing prana – our life force – to flow more readily. By lengthening the spine, we make space between the vertebra to allow for twists, flexion and extension of the spine.

I feel it is very important to de-emphasize goal orientation in yoga instruction such as "reach for your toes," "press your heels to the ground in down dog," or "hook your elbow past the knee." As we makespace for the breath in proper alignment, we allow for those "goals" to be reached organically. They simply come to the practitioner one day or they don't. Either way, yoga is not a competition. This minimizes frustration and self-criticism by simply *being* in yoga. What a lovely space this is.

Yoga is not a one-size-fits-all practice. As Patanjali laid out for us centuries ago, a teacher must teach to the student according to their abilities and resources available. Really Real Yoga places emphasis on observing the class at all times. By providing relief from the struggles of their asana practice, a yoga teacher enables all of the class to participate.

The teacher must learn to make the postures accessible to their students. Child's pose is not a suitable time out for yoga practitioners! I emphasize the use of straps, blocks, blankets, bolsters, chairs and a wall or railing to enable every student to feel the intended action within the pose. Others are provided alternative poses, modifications or alternative movements to bring blood flow to the space, increased flow of synovial fluid to the joints, length to the connective tissue, and enhanced breath to the practitioner.

The farther away from the spine, the more options we have with instruction to enable our students to be in the pose. By teaching people – not poses – we provide much more individual instruction within a group setting. When one feels like they are participating in more of the class, they enter a positive feedback loop of effort and reward. This encourages greater effort as obstacles fall away. Real yoga is applied at the individual level, yet when we share in a very good practice together, we experience an energy flow that transcends the individual. We know when it's special.

In the area of the spine are located the seven main chakras. While many people may focus on the colors, number of petals representative of each chakra, and seed sound of each, it is important to understand how the energies that are stored and managed in the area of the spine develop. Our spine is a storehouse of potential energy just by the way it is constructed. The events of our lives – to whom we were born and how we live – are contained within these domains of potential energy. Our emotional and intellectual levels, our social and private lives, are contained and reflected within our chakras (as well as other locations in our bodies). Study of the chakras provides an understanding of our emotional intelligence and development of self-awareness. This helps us to better relate with ourselves and with others.

As obstacles fall away in our physical practice, it allows for opening of awareness of the more subtle aspects of our lives – the subtle sheaths or the Kosha bodies. We spend time developing an understanding of how pranayama, chanting and mantras can lead to deeper levels of meditation. As this progresses, we gain a deeper awareness of how this healing focus provides insight into our being. What's important? What's not important?

We come to learn that by nourishing the more subtle aspects of our existence, we can be healthy and strong enough to serve others. With proper emphasis and focus on diet and exercise, on breath and life force, on minimizing thoughts that distract us or cause agitation, on being as present as possible in as many individual moments as possible, on thoughts and actions that take into consideration the welfare of others, we come to understand how we can continue on with expending energy in moments even when the physical body is tired. For it is the mental and spiritual levels of our existence that create this energy.

Where attention goes, energy flows. Where are we placing our thoughts and actions? Yoga helps us to understand this.

THE SKELETAL SYSTEM

THE STRUCTURE OF THE PHYSICAL BODY

To understand the skeletal system you must embrace this, "the foot bone is connected to the leg bone, the leg bone is connected to the hip bone ..." The skeleton, which weighs about 20 pounds, and works in partnership with the muscular system. Both systems are constantly renewing, and this renewal is essential, especially for bones. Without bone renewal, diseases such as osteoporosis may form. The skeletal system is not only the structure and support for our bodies, but it protects our organs. Thus, a strong skeleton is extremely important. In order to ensure a strong skeleton, one must remember and execute these three things – proper intake of protein, calcium and vitamins throughout life. One must exercise the skeletal system as well – it must be used to remain supple and strong.

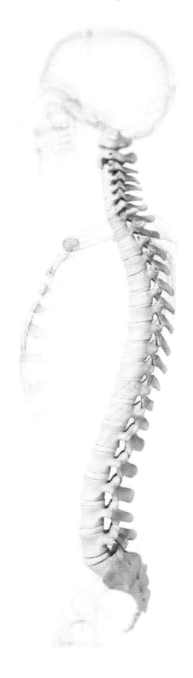

Axial Skeleton

The spine has twenty-four bones called vertebrae, which form the spinal column, and are divided into 3 major sections listed below.

• Cervical Spine has seven vertebrae which support your head's weight.

• Thoracic Spine has twelve vertebrae behind the chest to which the ribs are connected.

• Lumbar Spine has five vertebrae which support your body weight.

• The Sacrum is formed from five vertebrae fused into single bone that includes the coccyx.

The thoracic and sacral spines work to protect the major organs of the body while the cervical and lumbar spines help position the body weight over the legs. The sacral spine is part of the pelvic girdle.

The spine is used to support and transfer weight. The weight of the body must be transferred through the spine to the pelvic girdle through the legs and to the ground.

The front or anterior portion of the spine contains a kind of hydraulic system called intervertebral discs, acting somewhat like shock absorbers. They absorb shock, allow for some compression and are essential to movement. The back, or posterior section, is a complex of bony segments that protects the spinal cord. It also serves as the place for muscular attachments while forming joints with the ribs in the thoracic spine.

Appendicular Skeleton

The appendicular skeleton consists of the shoulder girdle and pelvic girdle. The shoulder girdle includes the arms and hands, and contains two paired bone segments – the scapula (shoulder blade) and clavicle (collarbone). The shoulder girdle and surrounding muscles control the movement of the arms. The pelvic area, which includes the legs, consists of two ball-and-socket joints formed by the right and left femurs. The pelvis is very strong and able to transfer weight from the pelvis to the rest of the joints in the leg, including the knees and ankles.

Bone Shapes

Bones have shapes and the shape of bones reflect their function.

• Long bones act as levers to raise and lower and help the body go deeper into postures.

• Short bones act as bridges and provide weight-bearing functions.

• Flat bones are very stable protective shells and a place for muscles to attach.

• Rounded bones are embedded with tendons.

• Irregular bones have peculiar form and include vertebrae, pelvis/ilium.

Joint Structure

Where two bones meet in the skeletal system is called a joint. Most joints are synovial joints, lubricated and mobile. They are attached by connective tissue that produce synovial fluid that circulates throughout the joint space. Bands of fibrous tissue called ligaments support and provide stability to the skeleton while allowing for mobility. They vary in size according to their function and they work to attach one bone to another at the joints. The skeleton contains many different types of joints; each form reflects its special function and determines the range of movement.

• Ball and socket joints, which are the most mobile, have a rounded head of one bone that fits into the socket of another bone. Examples – hips and shoulders.

• Hinge joints are the simplest of all joints and have great stability. The convex surface of one bone fits into the concave surface of another bone, allowing for flexion and extension. Examples – joints in fingers and knees.

• Pivot joints allow for rotation and have even greater stability. A pivot joint formed by the top of the cervical vertebrae allows the head to turn from side to side when you want to indicate "no." Example – vertebrae.

• Plane joints allow for gliding movements. Examples – some joints in the wrist and foot.

• Fixed joints are two bones that are almost fused together. Example – cranium.

DISEASES. DISORDERS. YOGA THERAPY.

WE BECOME WHAT WE EAT AND HOW WE LIVE; BODY, MIND, SOUL.

• Degeneration occurs naturally, simply caused by aging.

• Chronic stress is persistent stress and occurs when the body cannot process all the stressors in life.

• Fractures are broken bones.

• Accidents are unfortunate happenings that take place when one is not expecting it, often resulting in injury or harm to others.

• Joint pain is the stiffness in any joint and can be a sign of arthritis.

• Osteoporosis is the loss of bone density, which leads to an increased risk of bone fracture.

• Osteoarthritis is caused by the breakdown and eventual loss of the cartilage of one or more joints. Often affects ankles, knees, hips, fingers, wrists, elbows, shoulders, and the upper, middle and lower back.

• Rheumatoid arthritis is an autoimmune disease that causes chronic inflammation of the joints and surrounding tissue.

• Kyphosis is outward curve of the thoracic spine, also know as rounded back.

• Lordosis is inward curvature of the lumbar spine, just above the buttocks.

• Scoliosis is a sideways "C" or "S" shaped curve of the spine and is always abnormal.

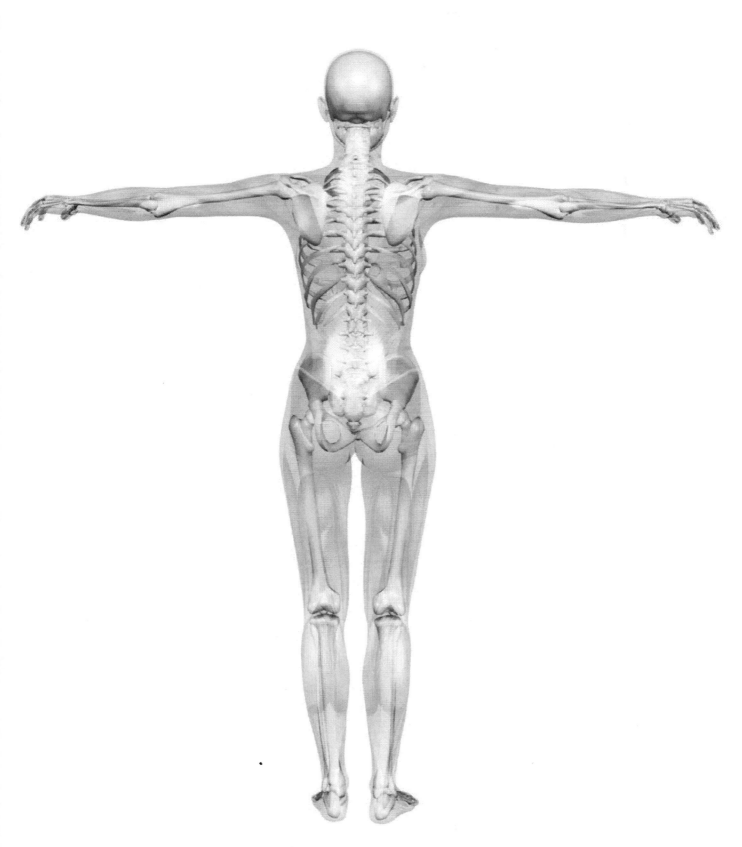

THE MUSCULAR SYSTEM

THE STRENGTH OF THE PHYSICAL BODY

The muscular system is often referred to as the machine of the body. This machine's main job is to provide us with movement and mobility. Though the human body itself is a complex mechanism, the muscles themselves work in a very simple way – they merely contract and relax. These actions are brought about by converting chemical energy into mechanical energy. The movement produced can be classified as either voluntary or involuntary. Within the muscular system there are three types of muscle tissues – cardiac, smooth and skeletal.

The cardiac muscles are one of the two types of involuntary muscles in our body and located only in the heart. These muscles are formed branching fibers and are controlled by impulses sent from the medulla oblongata of the brain.

The smooth muscles are the second grouping of involuntary muscles in our body. They make up our internal organs and aid in our digestion, circulation, urination, etc.

The skeletal muscles are the only voluntary muscles of our body. They are composed of long muscle fibers and show external mobility and movement in our bodies. These are the muscles we will focus on in the rest of this section. Skeletal muscles can be separated into groups based on their type of movement. This movement is built on the type of joint where the muscle is found. They generally act in pairs, one contracting while the other extends.

Flexors and Extensors – Bend at the joint/extend at the joint (i.e. biceps flex while triceps extend).

Abductors and Adductors – Pull away from the body/pull toward the body.

In the previous section of the skeletal system, a separation was made between the axial skeleton and the appendicular skeleton. The same division can be made with the muscular system as well.

Axial Muscles – The axial musculature arises on the axial skeleton and encompasses roughly 60 percent of the skeletal muscles. They are responsible for facial expression, eating and drinking, eye movements and all verbal communication. They are responsible for flexing, extending and rotating the head and neck in addition to the respiratory muscles. They also include the pelvic floor muscles, which comprise all movement in the openings and organs of the pelvic area.

Appendicular Muscles – The appendicular musculature stabilizes or moves parts of the appendicular skeleton and includes all skeletal muscles that are not classified as axial. This includes all the muscles within the shoulders, arms, hands, pelvis, legs and feet and makes up the remaining 40 percent of the skeletal muscles.

Lever Systems – Most body movement employs the mechanical principles of lever systems. A force of direction is applied to one part and the movement of weight is transferred elsewhere on that lever system. First class lever example – back of neck. Second class lever example – raising of heel. Third class lever example – flexing elbow.

Aerobic and Anaerobic – Aerobic exercise increases muscle endurance and strengthens the respiratory and cardiovascular systems. This includes activities such as hiking and swimming and involves longer lengths of consistent exercise. Anaerobic exercise causes enlargement of muscles and usually involves short, but intense exercise. This may included hiking quickly up a steep hill, weightlifting, or running a short distance very quickly.

Muscle Stretching – There are different types of muscle stretching but the majority of stretches are either dynamic or static.

• Static stretching, most common in yoga, involves no motion, affects static flexibility (and dynamic flexibility in some cases).
• Dynamic stretching involves motion and affects dynamic flexibility.
• Facilitated stretching involves lengthening the muscles, then contracting them, then lengthening them again to a new range of motion.

Muscle Contraction – Muscles produce movements. The way the muscles are shaped and how they are attached to the bone determine these movements. There are three types of muscle contraction –

• Concentric occurs when muscle shortens and moves a bone segment.
• Eccentric occurs when the muscle lengthens.
• Isometric (static) occurs when a muscle neither shortens nor lengthens, its contraction is simply held.

DISEASES. DISORDERS. YOGA THERAPY.
WE BECOME WHAT WE EAT AND HOW WE LIVE; BODY, MIND, SOUL.

• Common muscle strains and tears. Think RICE – Rest, Ice, Compression, Elevation. Rest the area, apply cold or heat and liniment oils. Acupuncture, massage and yoga can be very helpful.

• Repetitive strain injury. Rethink what is causing this injury and make lifestyle changes. Also, rest the area, apply cold or heat and liniment oils. Acupuncture, massage and yoga can be very helpful.

• Tenosynovitis and/or tendonitis is the inflammation of an area surrounding the tendon or the tendon itself.

• Soft-tissue inflammation is the swelling of a tendon.

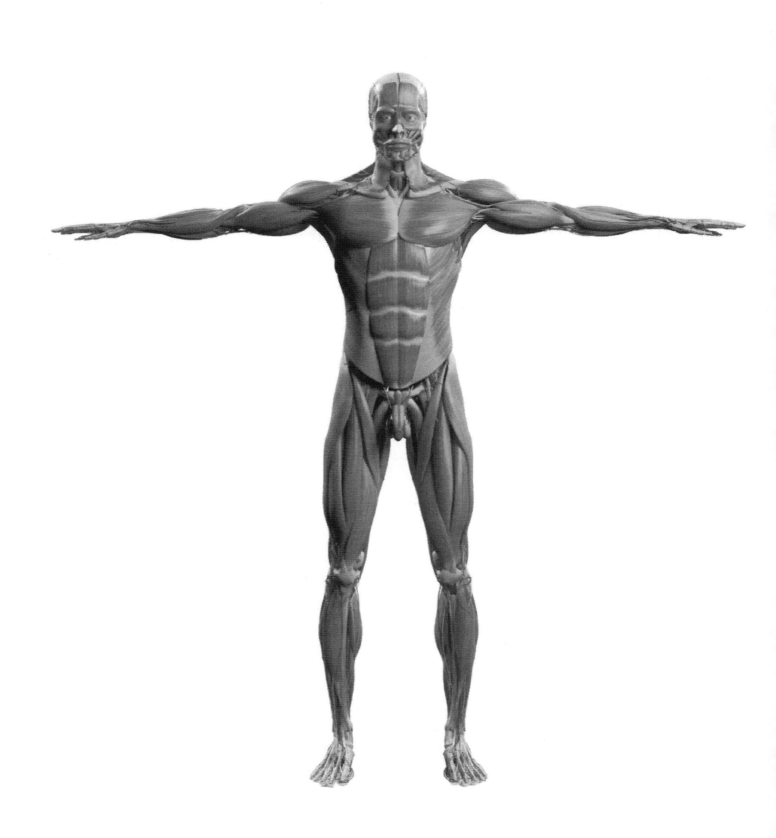

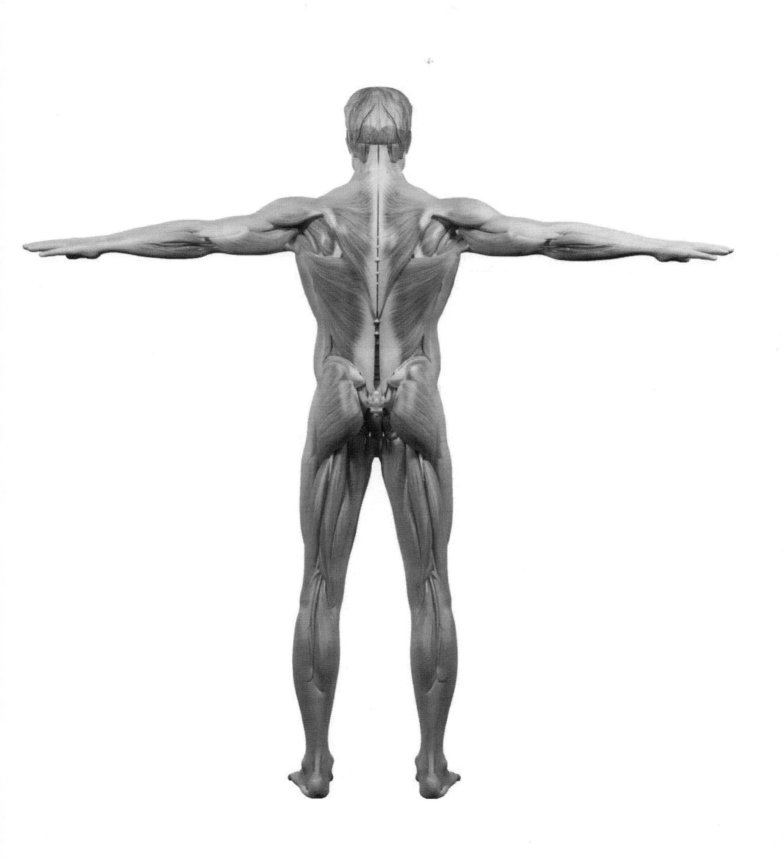

THE RESPIRATORY SYSTEM

ENJOY YOUR BREATH, IT IS A SIGN OF LIFE

From our first breath to our last, our bodies inhale oxygen and exhale carbon dioxide. It is with this process of respiration, along with the cardiovascular system, that our bodies are able to function. A normal breath rate ranges from 12-18 breaths per minute. However, a yogi's goal is to slow down the respiratory rate to about 8-12 breaths per minute. This is in order to develop the capacity to participate in demanding muscular activities with deeper and slower breaths. In order to fully understand your breathing patterns, you must fully understand the respiratory system. We must become aware of our breathing patterns in order to be physically and emotionally healthy. Breathing affects all parts of our body and can help us achieve greater stamina and muscle endurance while exercising. In order to achieve this, we need lifestyle adjustments, appropriate medical care, and yoga from a qualified teacher. Knowing how to breathe is essential; breathing is relaxing. When breathing patterns are deep, strong and slow, we have increased endurance, stamina and sense of well-being. Weak respiratory muscles, rigid and inelastic structures of the chest plus poor lung capacity often inhibit breathing. When breathing is impaired, the other systems of the body are negatively affected as well.

Three Part Breathing Process
The process by which oxygen is carried to body cells and carbon dioxide is carried away is called respiration. The upper part of the respiratory process warms and humidifies incoming air. The lower part provides space for the exchange of gases. This process generates energy cells that support and maintain bodily function.

- Pulmonary ventilation – the process of inhaling and exhaling.
- External respiration – the exchange of respiratory gases between lungs, the atmosphere and blood.
- Internal respiration – the exchange of respiratory gases between the blood and the body cells.

Respiratory Structure – From the nose to the lungs and back out again, air is filtered, heated and humidified. The respiratory system produces energy for the body tissues.

Nose – The nasal cavity is equipped with a sticky mucous membrane and nasal hairs that trap inhaled particles.

Voice Box – The larynx contains a leaf-shaped flap of cartilage that remains upright, allowing air to pass, but tips back and closes during swallowing so food does not enter the trachea. The vocal cords are fibrous bands that vibrate when air passes between them. Tighten the cords a little and low-pitched sounds are created. Tighten the cords a lot and high-pitched sounds are created.

Throat – The pharynx has three parts. The upper section allows air only to pass and the lower two sections allow food and liquids to pass.

Wind Pipes – The trachea, the main airway to the lungs, splits into two large branches to form an intricate root-like system in both the right and left lung.

Air Passages – The bronchi branch into smaller airways within both the right and left lung.

Lungs – The lungs are divided into lobes. The left lung has two lobes, the right lung has three.

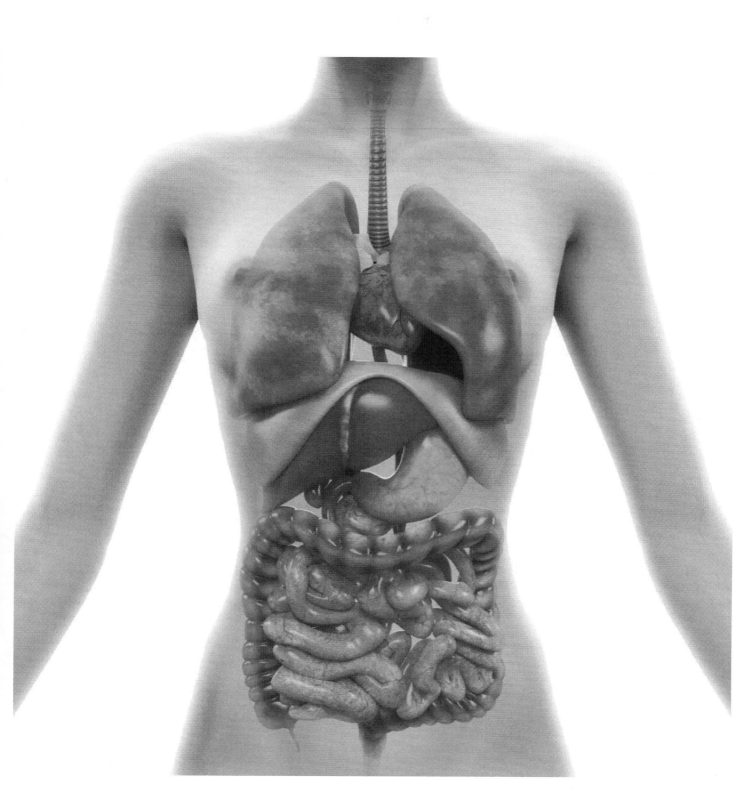

DISEASES. DISORDERS. YOGA THERAPY.

WE BECOME WHAT WE EAT AND HOW WE LIVE; BODY, MIND, SOUL.

Respiratory disorders are most commonly caused by infections. Lifestyle and environment are also important factors in keeping the respiratory system healthy.

• Upper airway infections affect the nasal sinuses, pharynx and larynx.

• Sinusitis is an infection in the air-filled cavities in the eye and nose area.

• Allergic asthma is an inflammation of the airways and lungs. Shortness of breath, a dry cough, even wheezing can occur. Household dust, animal dander and environmental pollution can play a part.

• Common cold has about 200 strains that are passed from person to person. How frequent are an individual's colds?

• Nosebleeds are blood running from the nostrils.

• Productive cough is a cough that extracts mucus from the respiratory tract.

• Tuberculosis is an infectious disease that can affect any tissue in the human body.

• Influenza is a viral infection that should be taken seriously. Symptoms include chills, fever, muscle pain, headache, weakness and cough.

• Bronchitis is an infection in the bronchi airways that join the windpipes to the lungs. Inflamed and swollen airways narrow and can cause mucus and cough.

• Pneumonia is usually caused by a bacterial infection, but sometimes caused by viruses. Symptoms include coughing, breathlessness, fever, joint and muscle pain.

THE CARDIOVASCULAR SYSTEM

LIFE REALLY IS AN INWARD JOURNEY TO YOUR SPIRITUAL HEART

Our hearts are the engines transporting goods through our blood on the tracks of our arteries, veins and capillaries. Without this very efficient transportation system, our bodies could not function. We would never receive nourishment from our digestive system, oxygen from our respiratory system, or hormones from our endocrine system. But this transportation system does not travel only one way; it's multifunctional. Waste and toxins are constantly extracted through this system and carried to the organs of elimination.

Our cardiovascular system, though extremely proficient, isn't immune to outside influences. Eating habits, daily activity and state of mind play an important role in its performance. Merely look at the effects fear or anxiety has on our heart rate to see how outside force can impact our bodies. Studies have uncovered the physiological and psychological benefits provided to this system by the practice of yoga. It appears to function more efficiently, showing greater stamina and aerobic power, improved circulation, lowered systolic and diastolic blood pressure, and decreased heart rate.

Pulmonary and Systemic Blood Circulation – The cardiovascular system is composed of two distinct circulatory paths – pulmonary and systemic blood circulation. Pulmonary circulation is where blood becomes oxygenated, and systemic cirulation is when the blood is circulated throughout the body.

Pulmonary Blood Circuit – The pulmonary blood circuit is the process through which the blood is oxygenated as it passes through the heart. De-oxygenated enters the heart through the superior vena cava and is pumped through the right ventricle and atrium, and to the lungs and capillaries, where carbon dioxide is exchanged for oxygen in the blood. Capillaries are extremely small vessels located within the tissues of the body that transport blood from the arteries to the veins. The blood then passes back into the heart which completes the pulmonary blood circuit. To the left ventricle and atrium, up through the aorta. From the aorta, oxygen-rich blood is then distrubuted throughout the body.

Systemic Blood Circuit – Once oxygenated blood re-enters the heart from the lungs, it passes through the left atrium and ventricle, up through the aorta. From the aorta, oxygen-rich blood is distributed throughout the body through a system of arteries and blood vessels. Once the oxygen stores of the blood are depleted, it is transferred in capillaries to veins throughout the body, which pass the blood through a system of one-way valves back to the superior vena cava.

Arteries – Carry oxygenated blood away from the heart and throughout the body.

Veins – Carry deoxygenated blood to the heart to become oxygenated again.

Heart – The beat of one's heart is an automatic occurrence about seventy times per minute. The heart and its surrounding areas work like a pump and a valve. The heart is able to pump blood so proficiently because there are two separate circulatory circuits with the heart as their common link. The heart pumps carry oxygenated and deoxygenated blood flow through the four heart chambers. The four heart valves allow for a one-way flow of blood through the heart.

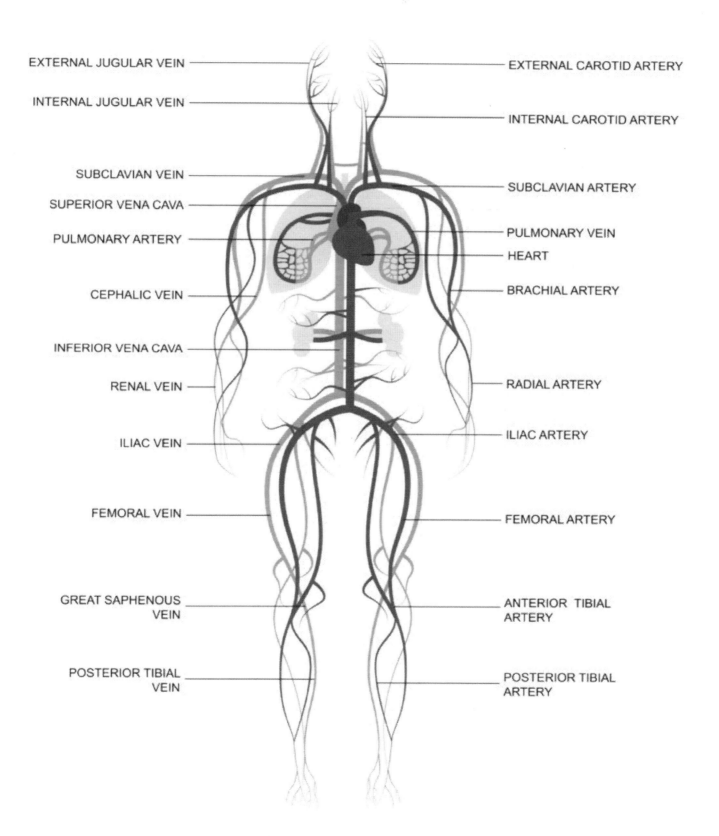

EXTERNAL JUGULAR VEIN

INTERNAL JUGULAR VEIN

SUBCLAVIAN VEIN

SUPERIOR VENA CAVA

PULMONARY ARTERY

CEPHALIC VEIN

INFERIOR VENA CAVA

RENAL VEIN

ILIAC VEIN

FEMORAL VEIN

GREAT SAPHENOUS
VEIN

POSTERIOR TIBIAL
VEIN

EXTERNAL CAROTID ARTERY

INTERNAL CAROTID ARTERY

SUBCLAVIAN ARTERY

PULMONARY VEIN

HEART

BRACHIAL ARTERY

RADIAL ARTERY

ILIAC ARTERY

FEMORAL ARTERY

ANTERIOR TIBIAL
ARTERY

POSTERIOR TIBIAL
ARTERY

DISEASES. DISORDERS. YOGA THERAPY.

WE BECOME WHAT WE EAT AND HOW WE LIVE; BODY, MIND, SOUL.

Cardiovascular system disorders are among the leading causes of poor health in the world.

• Unusual heartbeats and arrhythmia, when the heartbeat is abnormally slow, fast or irregular.

• Atherosclerosis is the narrowing of the arteries from a buildup of fat, cholesterol and plaque.

• Angina is chest pain that comes on with exertion and is a result of the heart not receiving sufficient oxygen in the blood.

• Heart attack the stopping of blood flow to the heart, usually causing part of the heart musule to die.

• Heart valve disorder is when one or more of the four valves are operating insufficiently.

• Heart murmurs are caused when the blood in the heart can be heard due to structural defects.

• Hypertension is persistent abnormally elevated blood pressure, a.k.a. high blood pressure.

THE DIGESTION & ELIMINATION SYSTEMS

LET THAT SHIT GO

Even before the first bite of food, the fantastic voyage of our digestive process has begun. Food is our fuel, but it has a long journey ahead of itself before it finishes its complete process. There are five primary functions of our digestive system that a simple piece of food will go through. Each of these functions is important to keep us healthy and when our digestion is strong, we have more energy, sounder sleep and have a higher resistance to disease.

First our food is ingested. It is broken down in the mouth by the teeth, tongue and jaw. Next, our food is digested and broken down further with acids, enzymes and buffers produced by the digestive tract. Then the food rests in the stomach and intestines, where it is churned and mixed. It then experiences absorption where the nutrients, which have been broken down during the digestion process, are moved into fluid that nourishes the cells of the body. Assimilation soon follows, during which nutrients of the cells are used by the body. And finally, it undergoes elimination in which indigestible waste is purged from the body through respiration, perspiration, urination and defecation.

Stool assessment, while seemingly awkward and strange, is important and an accurate way to monitor the health of our digestive systems. A healthy stool should be brown to light-brown; formed, but not hard, cylindrical and lacking a strong odor. While proper bowel movements are important, our urinary system is also vital in eliminating waste from the body. This system regulates mineral concentrations in the blood along with blood volume and pressure. It also helps the body detoxify and works with the lungs, skin and intestines to keep the chemicals and water in our bodies balanced.

Mouth, Teeth, Tongue – Work to break down food so it can travel into the body.

Salivary Glands – Secrete saliva in your mouth.

Jaw – Works with the above to chew and break down food.

Pharynx – Or throat squeezes and propels food down the esophagus.

Esophagus – A muscular tube that carries food and saliva from the mouth to the stomach.

Stomach – Secretes gastric juices that further break down food; is roughly the size of your fist.

Liver – Produces substances that break down fats.

Gall Bladder – Stores bile, which emulsifies fats and neutralizes acids in partly digested food.

Pancreas – Produces enzymes that break down digestible foods.

Small Intestine – The most extensive part of digestion occurs here; most food products are absorbed.

Large Intestine – Responsible for absorption of water and excretion of solid waste materials.

Rectum – Acts as a temporary storage facility for feces.

Kidneys – Act as a filter, removing urea from the blood through tiny filtering units called nephrons. Urine then travels through two long thin tubes called ureter.

Ureter – Muscles in the ureter walls constantly tighten and relax to force urine downward and away from the kidneys. The urine then empties into the bladder.

Bladder and Urethra – Store urine until you are ready to empty it. A healthy bladder can hold about 16 ounces of urine for 2 to 5 hours comfortably. Urine leaves the body through the urethra.

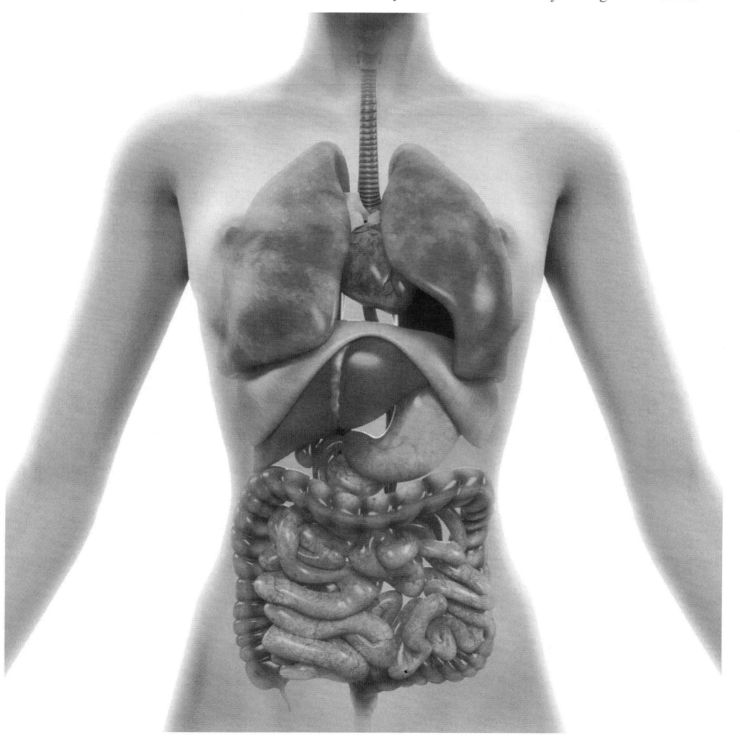

DISEASES. DISORDERS. YOGA THERAPY.

WE BECOME WHAT WE EAT AND HOW WE LIVE; BODY, MIND, SOUL.

The Digestive System

Digestive system disorders occur more frequently than other illnesses and can affect people of any age.

• Acidity is a sharp burning sensation in the lower chest just below the sternum, often caused by overeating, drinking or use of drugs – even aspirin.

• Indigestion is associated with abdominal pain, nausea, vomiting, belching, acidity or gas.

• Constipation is a sign that waste from the bowels have not completely emptied from the body.

• Diarrhea is the sudden onset of frequent watery stools associated with abdominal infection.

• Irritable bowel syndrome is a combination of abdominal pain and altered bowel function due to disturbances in the large intestines. Low fiber diet, use of laxatives or stress brings this on.

The Urinary System

Urinary system disorders occur when the kidneys are unable to filter out waste from the blood.

• Incontinence is the involuntary loss of urine from the bladder. Common with the elderly due to loss of muscle strength of the pelvic floor, stroke or loss of control of the nervous system.

• Frequent urination is the constant urge to urinate.

• Painful urination is pain, burning or discomfort when urinating.

• Blood in urine is a sign of trauma, kidney stones or even cancer.

THE NERVOUS SYSTEM

IT IS THE JOB OF THE SPINE TO KEEP THE BRAIN ALERT

The nervous system coordinates and controls everything in the body. It is responsible for sending, receiving and processing nerve impulses which enable the movement of our muscles, monitor the function of our organs, assemble the input from our senses, and initiate our direct responses and actions. This system is often divided into the Central Nervous System (CNS) and the Peripheral Nervous System (PNS). The CNS, consisting of the brain and spinal cord, represents the largest part of our nervous system. The PNS encompasses all other nerves and neurons not found within the CNS.

While the Central Nervous System is customarily considered one structure, the PNS can be subdivided into the Sensory-Somatic Nervous System (SSNS) and the Autonomic Nervous System (ANS). The SSNS, consisting of the neurons connected with the skin, muscles and sense organs, is considered the link between our surroundings, such as what we may hear, see or feel, and our CNS. Sensory neurons carry nerve impulses from a given sense organ, such as our fingertips when touching something hot, to our CNS. The motor neurons would then carry nerve impulses away from the CNS to our muscles, causing us to pull away from the heated source. This example demonstrates how the SSNS is associated with voluntary control of our body movements.

Central Nervous System (CNS) – Consists of the brain and the spinal cord. The CNS processes all sensory data and motor commands and is responsible for intelligence, learning, memory and emotion. The brain receives sensory input from the spinal cord as well as from its own nerves. The spinal cord is an extension of the brain. The spinal cord connects a large part of the Peripheral Nervous System to the brain. Information (nerve impulses) reaches the spinal cord through the sensory neurons.

Peripheral Nervous System (PNS) – Consists of the neural tissue surrounding the CNS. It provides sensory information to the CNS and carries motor commands throughout the body. The PNS can be divided into the SSNS and ANS.

Sensory Somatic Nervous System (SSNS) – Consists of 12 pairs of cranial nerves and 31 pairs of spinal nerves. This system emerges from the CNS to form part of the PNS. The sensory nerves perform sensory and motor functions. The 12 cranial nerves perform mainly head and neck functions. The 31 spinal nerves emerge from the spinal cord and extend through the vertebrae. Each pair of nerves subdivides into a number of branches allowing for movement throughout the body.

Autonomic Nervous System (ANS) – Pimarily involved in the unconscious control of our bodies, the ANS is responsible for maintaining our internal balance and responding to changes in the environment. This includes heart rate, blood pressure, respiration, digestion, salivation, metabolism, perspiration, excretion and temperature. This does not mean that this system isn't involved with any voluntary actions. Some of its functions work along with the conscious mind, such as in the case of breathing. The ANS can be further divided into the sympathetic nervous system, parasympathetic nervous system and enteric nervous system. The sympathetic and parasympathetic nervous systems generally work in complementary opposition to each other. The first by and large serves in inciting quick responses, whereas the second stimulates that which doesn't require immediate reactions. It's "flight or fight" versus "rest and digest." The enteric nervous system is the part of the nervous system that manages the digestive functions of our gastrointestinal tract, pancreas and gall bladder. Some medical professionals believe there is an important relationship between the enteric nervous system and our immune system.

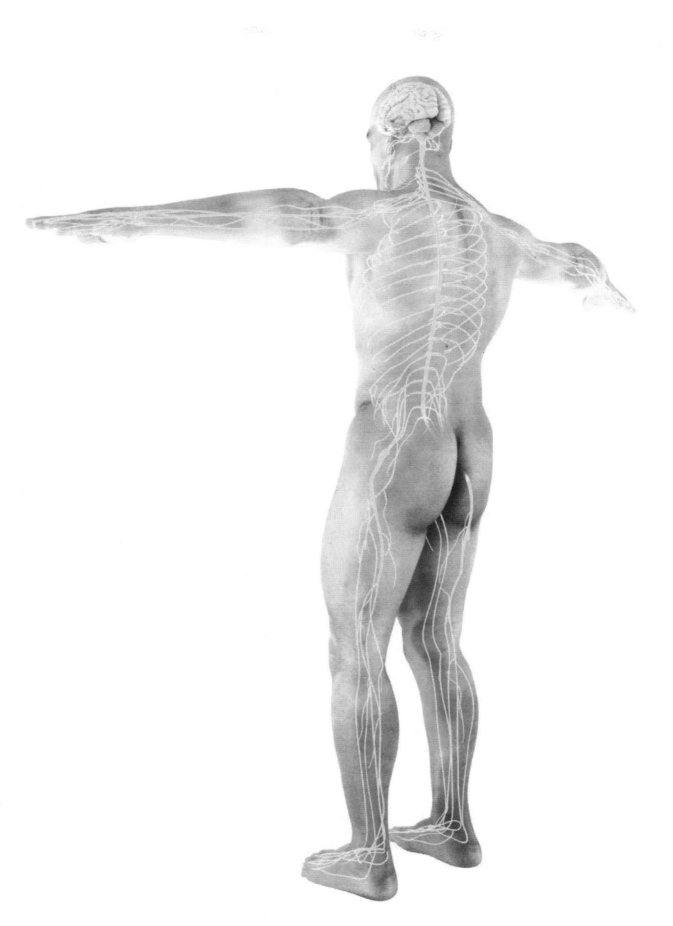

DISEASES. DISORDERS. YOGA THERAPY.

WE BECOME WHAT WE EAT AND HOW WE LIVE; BODY, MIND, SOUL.

Nervous system disorders can impair both physical and mental function. If electrical impulses in the brain or spinal cord are not working properly, disorders can occur. Damage to the spinal cord can cause loss of sensation in some parts of the body or mind, even causing paralysis.

• Migraines or simple headaches can cause pain, dizziness, visual problems, even nausea.

• Eye strain or visual problems such as glaucoma are the eyes' inability to focus. The disturbance can lead to permanent sight loss.

• Epilepsy is abnormal brain activity and can cause uncontrollable seizures.

• The sciatica nerve is the largest in your body. Sciatic pain can run from the lower spine down both legs to the feet.

• Multiple sclerosis is caused by the body's immune system attacking its own tissues, affecting movement, vision, speech and other functions.

• Parkinson's disease is a degenerative condition that affects nerves in the brain, causing stiffness and trembling of the muscles, and interfering with walking, speech and facial expressions.

• Dementia is the deterioration of mental ability due to brain disease. The most common form is Alzheimer's disease. Small brain blockages can even cause a stroke.

• Stroke is damage to the brain due to blockage of blood supply, resulting in lack of oxygen.

• Paralysis is damage to the brain or spinal cord resulting in loss of activity in the damaged path of that nerve.

• Loss of hearing can occur either due to defects, drugs or loud noise in excess.

• Blackouts are temporary losses of memory or consciousness.

• Seizures are sudden attacks or spasm of the muscles.

• General numbness or tingling is when limbs are deprived of the ability to move or feel.

• Loss of balance is the disruption of equilibrium in the body.

THE ENDOCRINE SYSTEM

YOU HAVE THE POWER TO CREATE OPTIMAL BALANCE IN YOUR LIFE

The glands of the endocrine system influence almost every cell, organ and function of our bodies through the release of over 20 major hormones into blood vessels, which circulate by way of the bloodstream. These hormones alter the metabolism of their target organ can increase or decrease its activity. Though we seldom consider this system in relation to our overall health, it plays a significant role in regulating our mood, growth, development, metabolism and the functions of our tissues, sexual life and reproductive system.

In order to keep our endocrine system and, in turn, ourselves healthy, we must pay close attention to any and all stress on our bodies as hormones have a very influential impact on our physical, intellectual and emotional behavior. The effects of stress can manifest in many ways, and most all of them are influenced by our endocrine system. We may find ourselves plagued with weight, memory or sleep issues. It may affect our digestion, blood pressure or cholesterol. We can even experience sexual dysfunction or immune system problems. These examples alone demonstrate how stress of virtually any nature may well be at the core of our health issues.

In most cases, problems with our endocrine system can be reversed. Relaxation, meditation and yoga can help to ease the pressures of our daily grind. Paying close attention to our diet and food-related behaviors can aid in weight or digestion issues. Anything to get our mind off the stressors of our lives can be very beneficial to our physical and emotional well-being. The role of the endocrine system is to respond to our stressors, get the stress levels under control, and restore balance to the system.

The Endocrine System consists of seven major glands, each with a corresponding chakra.

Pineal Gland – Releases melatonin, which influences the body's physiological rhythms – linked to day/night cycles of the body and sexual development. The seventh chakra links to this organ.

Pituitary Gland – Releases hormones that regulate the other glands and their functions along with their metabolic processes. The hormones it releases stimulate the thyroid and adrenal glands, regulate the gonads, and stimulate mammary glands and the uterus. It also releases growth hormone and can be considered the growth gland. The sixth chakra links to this organ.

Thyroid and Parathyroid Gland – Increase our ability to use energy and oxygen. They produce hormones that affect bones, kidneys and intestines while regulating calcium in our body fluids. This influences the growth of the skeletal system. The fifth chakra links to this organ.

Thymus Gland – Releases hormones that target defense cells, which influence the strength of our immune system. The fourth chakra links to this organ.

Pancreas – Has two separate functions via the exocrine and endocrine glands. Exocrine gland secretes digestive enzymes that break down carbohydrates, fats and proteins. Endocrine gland, a.k.a. energy gland, produces glucagon and insulin, which regulate blood sugar levels. The third chakra links to this organ.

Gonads – The male and female reproductive organs. Testosterone is released from testes. Estrogen and progesterone is released from ovaries. These hormones promote production and growth of sperm and eggs, along with influencing male and female behavioral patterns. The second chakra links to this organ.

Adrenal Gland – Sometimes referred to as the energy gland. Releases hormones that affect metabolic and regulatory functions in the cells. This gland secretes epinephrine and norepinephrine, which increase cardiac activity and blood pressure. This gland is responsible for the "adrenaline rush" you sometimes feel. The first chakra links to this organ.

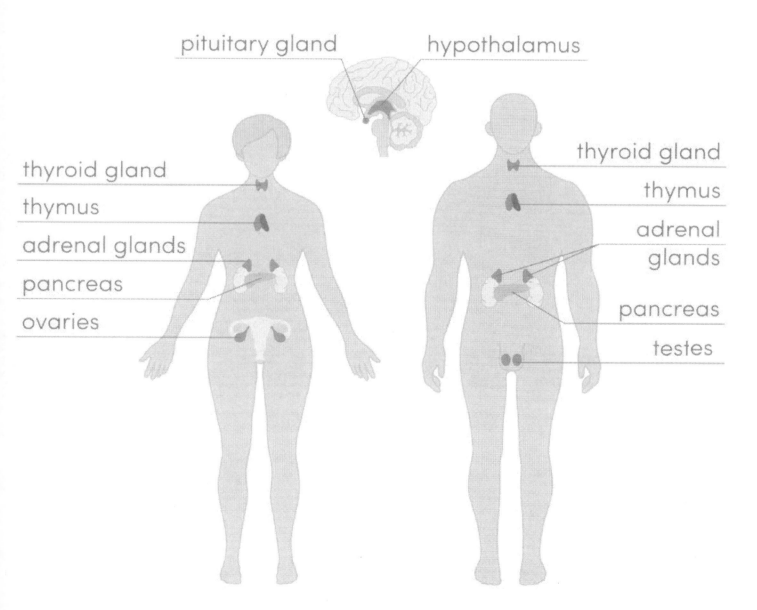

DISEASES. DISORDERS. YOGA THERAPY.

WE BECOME WHAT WE EAT AND HOW WE LIVE; BODY, MIND, SOUL.

• Stress is a specific response by the body that interferes with the normal equilibrium of an organism.

• Fatigue is weariness from exertion.

• Depression is a condition of emotional withdrawal.

• Weakened immune systems can be caused by many things ranging from the common cold and influenza to the more serious like cancer and AIDS.

• Diabetes I – the pancreas is incompetent at producing insulin, which regulates the sugar levels in the body. This is genetic.

• Diabetes II – the pancreas produces insulin, but the body no longer responds normally to the insulin. This is also known as "insulin resistance" and is the type of diabetes developed over time due to diet and lifestyle. (Excessive thirst may be a sign of diabetes.)

THE LYMPHATIC SYSTEM
HOLDING ON TO ANGER, WORRY, JEALOUSY AND WHAT OTHERS THINK IS JUST A WASTE OF TIME

The lymphatic system is our body's basic defense mechanism. The main function of the system is the making, maintaining, and allocating of special cells. These cells are vital for the body's defense system. It also aids in the delivery of nutrients and the extraction of wastes from the bloodstream, while working to maintain the normal blood volume.

Lymph Fluid – An almost colorless fluid that travels through vessels in the lymphatic system and carries cells that help fight infection and disease.

Immunity – There are two main types of immunity – innate immunity and naturally acquired immunity. A third is that of active immunization, when the body is intentionally introduced to a pathogen in the form of a vaccine.

• Innate immunity is present at birth. An example of this is the body's response to a cut that is infected; the innate immunity produces the pus.

• Naturally acquired immunity emerges after the body's exposure following an introduction of a particular pathogen.

Lacrimal Gland – A small almond-shaped structure in the eye that produces tears, which protect the eyes.

Subclavian Veins and Thoracic Duct – Lymph drains from the upper right part of the body into the right subclavian vein while lymph from the rest of the body collects in the Thoracic Duct, draining into the left subclavian vein.

Tonsils and Adenoids – Filter germs that attempt to invade the body and help to develop antibodies.

Thymus Gland – Location where T-cells, also known as lymphocytes, mature.

Spleen – Purifies the contents of the blood through production of antibodies and filtration of damaged red blood cells.

Cisterna Chyli – Lymph from the lower body converge to form this vessel.

Nodes – Filter the lymphatic fluid and store special cells that can trap cancer cells or bacteria that are traveling through the body in the lymph fluid. Note – Nodes are found throughout the body.

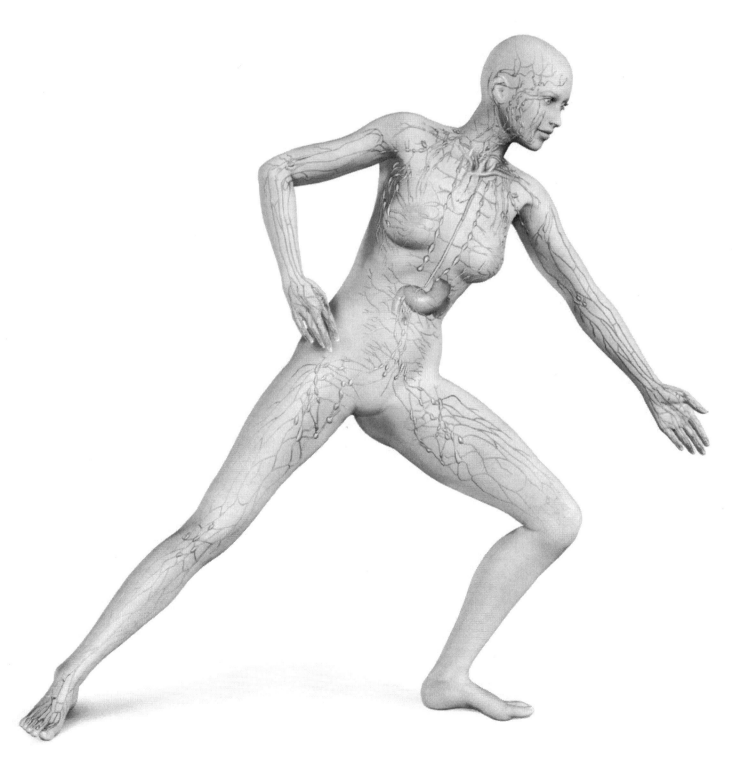

DISEASES. DISORDERS. YOGA THERAPY.

WE BECOME WHAT WE EAT AND HOW WE LIVE; BODY, MIND, SOUL.

The immune system produces antibodies to fight infections and sometimes to prevent reinfection. There are two types of immune system disorders –

(1) The Immune system overreacts.

• Allergies produce an overabundance of histamine in reaction to otherwise harmless substances (pollen, animal dander, fragrances).

• Autoimmune disorders – the immune system forms antibodies, not against invaders, but against the body's own tissue.

(2) The immune system is too weak to deal with threats to health including stress.

• Chronic Fatigue Syndrome (CFS) – when the immune system is too weak to deal with stress.

• HIV destroys a specific type of white blood cells, rendering the immune system less effective and the body more susceptible to disease. As cell numbers fall, the immune system becomes less and less effective, causing AIDS.

• Chronic infections are infections in which the pathogens create equilibrium with the body, making the infection present for long periods of time.

• Enlarged lymph nodes may be a sign of an infection or something more serious, such as cancer.

THE FIVE BODIES
EACH A LITTLE MORE TRANSPARENT THAN THE ONE BEFORE

JUST AS A MAN CASTS OFF WORN OUT CLOTHES AND PUTS ON NEW ONES

SO ALSO THE EMBODIED SELF CASTS OFF WORN OUT BODIES ~ BHAGAVAD GITA, 2.22

By understanding the subtleties of the three bodies and the five sheaths within the three bodies, one has the ability to better understand the importance of the yoga asanas as a means to unify the Self. Through a sincere practice, communication of the external towards the internal Self is developed. As unification develops between the bodies, a total being toward a conscious Soul arises.

Anatomical Sheath – Annamaya Kosha – Our densest layer, where yoga exploration begins.
The physical body is born, grows, changes, decays and then dies. Proper care of the physical body is necessary for nourishment and growth. Proper food and asanas aid in this growth.

Life Force Sheath – Pranamaya Kosha – Altered states of energetics using breath regulation.
The astral body is connected to the physical body by a subtle thread through which vital currents pass. The astral body contains the prana, or life force energy, the mind, the intellect and the emotions. It is comprised of layers, each one more subtle that the one before.

Mental Sheath – Manomaya Kosha – Our fluctuating mental and emotional layer.
The mental/emotional body encompasses our ego/personality. This is where our fluctuating thoughts and feelings reside, making this body perhaps the most important body for the development of our being. Meditation helps illuminate awareness, leading to personal growth and joy in living.

Intellectual Sheath – Vijnanamaya Kosha – Awareness, beyond thought, observation, witness.
The seat of our witnessing consciousness, steady and constant, this body is transformed by studying the scriptures with sincerity.

Bliss Sheath – Anandamaya Kosha – Love, Joy, Peace, Freedom.
In Sanskrit, "karana sharira" is better known as the seed body. Just as a seed bulb contains within itself everything needed to sprout and grow, the seed body stores subtle impressions in the form of karma. Karma is not fate, destiny or luck; it is a result of your own past actions. Everything that has happened to you in this life and in past lives is stored here. These subtle impressions control the formation and growth of the other bodies and determine the aspects of the next birth. At the time of death, the astral body and the causal body, which remain together, separate from the physical body. To return to this harmonized state is to return to our true nature.

THE NADIS OF THE ENERGETIC BODY
LIFE IS A BALANCE OF HOLDING ON AND LETTING GO

IN ORDER TO BE TRUTHFUL

YOU MUST EMBRACE YOUR TOTAL BEING ~ RUMI

The Nadis of the Energic Body
Nadis are essentially channels of energy. They compose the subtle body, circulating vital life force or prana, from the crown of your head to the tips of your toes. In Eastern philosophy, the nadis are often thought to influence a person's health, be it physical, mental, emotional or spiritual. When the energies are in a state of balance, the body, mind and spirit function in harmony, rendering good health in the individual.

If the flow is disrupted, energies suffer an imbalance. The body, mind and spirit no longer act in harmony; instead they begin to operate in discord, which can lead to disease. This isn't the traditional definition of disease, though an imbalance in the flow of energy can cause illness. It's also in reference to the feelings of vitality, bliss, strength and inner peace. An imbalanced flow of energy can cause lethargy, misery, weakness and inner unrest or turmoil. It is not uncommon for people to experience an alternating dominance of one nadi over another, even throughout the course of a day, which can result in issues with personality and behavior as well as health.

The number of nadis that flow through the body varies from text to text. Some scriptures cite upwards of 72,000 nadis, while other teachings maintain that there are only 14. But regardless of where you draw your information, most texts agree that three of the nadis are by far the most important – Sushumna, Ida and Pingala.

Main Nadis – Sushumana
Sushumna is the main nadi or channel of energy. It's said to run the entire length of the spinal cord, starting at the base of the spine and flowing up to the crown of the head. Along its upward path, Sushumna comes into contact with each of the seven chakras. Actually, Sushumna begins in the root chakra, or muladhara, and is thought to end at the crown chakra, or sahasrara, the thousand-petalled lotus. It is for this reason that Sushumna nadi is believed to be the path of enlightenment for the subtle body.

Moon Nadis – Ida
Beginning and ending on the left side of Sushumna is Ida or the moon nadi. It revolves around the main nadi, passing through each of the chakras. It's said to be the feminine nadi, since it's considered nurturing in nature. As energy flows through Ida nadi, the body and the mind are both nurtured and purified. People experiencing a dominance of Ida nadi may tend to nurture and greatly care for others, but can lack the strength to sustain a strong yoga practice. The potential is there, yet without a balance in Pingala, they may remain stunted in both the material and spiritual worlds.

Sun Nadis – Pingala
Beginning and ending on the right side of Sushumna is Pingala or the sun nadi. It too revolves around the main nadi, passing through each of the chakras. It's said to be the masculine nadi, since it's considered vital in nature. As energy flows through Pingala nadi, it also purifies the body and mind, but this cleansing is like fire. People suffering a dominance of Pingala nadi tend to be filled with creativity and energy, but without a balance in Ida, they may not reflect or ponder things enough to achieve spiritual wealth.

THE SEVEN CHAKRAS

WHERE ATTENTION GOES ENERGY FLOWS

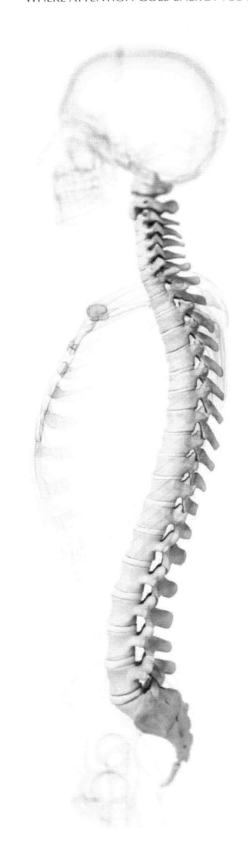

THE SEVEN CHAKRAS

THE MIND IS THE MASTER OF THE SENSES, AND THE BREATH IS THE MASTER OF THE MIND ~ B.K.S. IYENGAR

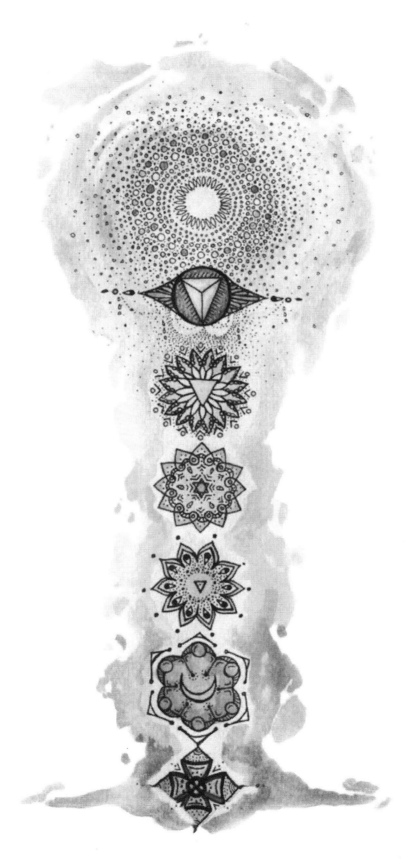

FIRST CHAKRA — ROOT CHAKRA — MULADHARA

ROOT SOLID AND REACH UPWARD TO A HIGHER AWARENESS OF YOUR TRUE SELF

Our first chakra is often described as our root chakra and the foundation of our subtle system. It is this chakra that acts as a driving force to keep us grounded and centered. When neglected, a person may find themselves unfocused and almost drifting through life. They may experience moments of fear, uncertainty and frustration. In turn, when this chakra is developed and nurtured, a person will discover a certain sense of security, confidence and satisfaction. The will to love and enjoy life is one of the greatest signs of optimum functioning of this chakra.

The most prominent quality of this chakra is innocence as it is the least complicated of our chakras. When we are born, every action or need is completely innocent. It is solely to fulfill our base needs such as food, clothing, shelter or community. It can be said we should find in us the wisdom of a child. As an adult, if we were to act or react from the basis of these necessities, our actions would hold no motive. They would be more altruistic in nature. Once our basic needs are met, we should, in theory, have everything we would ever want or desire in this world and need never act out of personal gain. We would have a balance, understanding the difference between want and need. Social influence, in general, tends to cloud this intrinsic innocence and shrouds the wisdom that comes with it.

Through meditation, we can learn to be more innocent in our needs, more selfless in our actions, and more enlightened in our path. We begin to see that all life is connected. Each choice we make influences the whole of life. If we have more, someone else must have less. Just watching the news alone should demonstrate this idea. Once we've nurtured this chakra and our needs are met, we should then be able to move forth to the creative nature of life, the building of our self-worth, and the strengthening of our intuition.

Muladhara Truths
• Sanskrit translation – root support
• Color – red
• Petals – 4
• Element – Earth
• Sound vibration, Bija Mantra – LAM
• Sense organ – nose, sense of smell
• Develops – in the womb, during birth, the first twelve months of life
• Location – perineum
• Physical body – legs, feet, skeletal system, immune system, large intestine, adrenals
• Physical imbalances – Irritable Bowel Syndrome (IBS), constipation, hemorrhoids, weight issues, arthritis, poor balance, foot or leg issues, lower back or sciatica
• Emotional imbalances – rigid, controlling, lacking imagination

Yoga Path
• Hatha

Tools
• Oils – Patchouli, Sandalwood, Vetiver, Ginger, Thyme, Basil
• Gems – Hematite, Garnet, Black Tourmaline, Smoky Quartz, Bloodstone, Ruby
• Incenses – Cedar, Sage, Patchouli

Tuning in With Breath
• Location
• Touch
• Contraction with Breath Retention

Tuning in With a Grounding Meditation
• Include the sound vibration "Lam" and the "Earth" element.

Asana Options
• Mountain
• Chair
• Tree
• Downward Facing Dog
• Staff
• Head to Knee
• Lotus
• Bound Angle
• Half Locust
• Full Locust
• Knees to Chest
• Bridge
• Savasana under blankets

Eating for This Chakra
Root vegetables – carrots, potatoes, parsnips, radishes, beets, onions, garlic, etc.

Protein-rich foods – eggs, meats, beans, tofu, tempeh, legumes, nuts, peanut butter.

Spices – horseradish, hot paprika, chives, cayenne, pepper.

Based on Chakra One, Please Answer the Following Questions

What do I accept as truths concerning my body? Survival? The Earth?

_____
_____
_____
_____
_____
_____
_____
_____
_____
_____

Is there an environment that nourishes me? Am I able to find it?

_____
_____
_____
_____
_____
_____
_____
_____
_____
_____

Do I respect and care for my body?

_____
_____
_____
_____
_____
_____
_____
_____
_____
_____

SECOND CHAKRA — SACRAL CHAKRA — SWADHISTHANA

MY POWER IS A NATURAL EXTENTION OF MY CREATIVITY

Our second chakra is often described as our sacral chakra and is considered the dwelling place of Self. It is this chakra that affords us the ability to move and change. Our place in this world is not to influence the relationships and things around us, but to be open and accept them as they are. We must learn to let go of our control. It is also this chakra that acts as the governing power behind the emotional and sensual aspects of our lives. If ignored, a person may become emotionally explosive, manipulative and resistant to change. Though the hardest chakra to heal, since its health is often linked to our upbringing, we can experience – when unobstructed – a flow of emotional, sensual and creative energy throughout our bodies. A feeling of balance is a good indication our second chakra has been nourished.

The most prominent quality of this chakra is creativity. As people began to understand their basic needs, the process by which to secure those needs was developed and made real. It is this simple idea that tells us creation resides within each of us. And without ego, we are all able to be inspired and be confident with this inspiration.

Proper balance in this chakra manifests our capacity to freely flow with our emotions and relate with those around us, yet still recognize that our self-worth is not based upon these factors. We begin to react to things intuitively, not thinking and weighing our options or finding ways to exploit the events in our paths. We act and react without ego, seeing things with thoughtless awareness.

Swadhisthana Truths
- Sanskrit translation – sacred home of Self
- Color – orange
- Petals – 6
- Element – water
- Sound vibration, Bija Mantra – VAM
- Sense organ – tongue, taste
- Develops – six months to two years
- Location – above genital and below navel, sacrum
- Physical body – blood, lymph, mucus, semen, urine, saliva, low back, womb, genitals, kidney, bladder, circulatory system
- Physical imbalances – breast and prostrate cancer, sexual issues
- Emotional Imbalances – depressed, seems to be impossible to make happy, no initiative, aggressive, manipulative, ascetic to the point of denying pleasure

Yoga Path
• Tantra

Tools
• Oils – Frankincense, Patchouli, Jasmine, Clary Sage, Sweet Marjoram, Cypress
• Gems – Moonstone, Tourmaline, Coral, Citrine, Pearl, Aquamarine, Clear Quartz
• Incenses – Cedarwood, Juniper

Tuning in With Breath
• Location
• Touch
• Contraction with Breath Retention

Tuning in With a Sweetness Meditation
• Include the sound vibration "Vam" and the "Water" element.

Asana Options
• Spinal Twists
• Reversed Plank
• Boat
• Crescent
• Goddess Squat
• Standing Hip Circles
• Bow
• Cowhead
• Bridge
• Pelvic Rock
• Reclining Goddess
• Reclining Scissor Kicks
• Plow
• Fish
• Savasana with hands on belly

Eating for This Chakra
Liquids – water, mineral water.

Fish & Seafood – salmon, tuna, shrimp, sardines, anchovies, oysters, scallops, etc.

Sweet fruits – melons, mangos, strawberries, passion fruit, oranges, coconut, etc.

Nuts – almonds, walnuts, cashews, etc.

Spices – cinnamon, vanilla, carob, sweet paprika, sesame seeds, caraway seeds.

Based on Chakra Two, Please Answer the Following Questions

Do I have comfort in and with my sexuality?

_____
_____
_____
_____
_____
_____
_____
_____
_____
_____

How do I feel about change?

_____
_____
_____
_____
_____
_____
_____
_____
_____
_____
_____
_____

Where or in what do I find my bliss? Am I able to appreciate this bliss?

_____
_____
_____
_____
_____
_____
_____
_____
_____
_____
_____

THIRD CHAKRA — NAVEL CHAKRA — MANIPURA

MY ACTIONS AND BEHAVIOR ARE MANIFESTED FROM THE CORE BELIEF THAT
MY AUTHENTIC SELF IS POWERFUL AND CAN MOVE ME TO ANY PLACE I DESIRE

Our third chakra is called our solar plexus or navel chakra and is the seat of intellect. It is this chakra that is the center of our personal power and is action oriented. If underdeveloped, a person will most likely carry with them a low self-esteem. They may have a tendency to lie, withdraw from obstacles, feel depressed, worry or lack confidence in the things they do from day to day. When this chakra is kept in balance, a person will find a clear sense of optimism or self-respect and the ability to fully express themselves or face new challenges with confidence. They will possess a strong sense of personal power.

The most prominent quality of this chakra is satisfaction. To truly nurture this chakra, we must recognize our personal path in life is only ours to walk. And there comes a time when we must take the emotional steps to grow from a child to an adult; not letting go of our dreams or aspirations, but taking action to make them real. We are blessed with an intellect and a body through which we can work to satisfy our basic needs. But there is a line where need becomes want that we do not want to cross. This should empower us to live our best lives and find a satisfaction in our actions toward our goals.

It is also believed that this is our intuitive chakra, where we can find our gut feelings that tell us to do or not do any given thing. If our self-esteem is lacking, our intuitive skills may not develop or we may not possess the confidence to listen to our gut. It is no wonder that this insight we all hold would be found at the center of our being. It is here that we can feel calm and peaceful.

Manipura Truths
- Sanskrit translation – shining gems
- Color – yellow
- Petals – 10
- Element – fire
- Sound vibration, Bija Mantra – RAM
- Sense organ – eyes, sight
- Develops – eighteen months to three years
- Location – at navel, solar plexus
- Physical body – digestive organs, pancreas, liver, gall bladder, adrenals
- Physical imbalances – digestive problems, food intolerances, muscle spasms, blood sugar oroblems, diabetes, eating disorders, paralysis
- Emotional imbalances – easiy manipulated or controlled by others, overabundant burnout, desire for fame, attention-seeking

Yoga Path
• Karma

Tools
• Oils – Chamomile, Bergamot, Juniper, Fennel, Peppermint
• Gems – Amber, Tiger's Eye, Yellow Topaz, Ruby, Green Jade, Blue Sapphire
• Incenses – Sandalwood, Nag Champa, Dragon's Blood Resin

Tuning in With Breath
• Location
• Touch
• Contraction with Breath Retention

Tuning in With a Empowerment Meditation
• Include the sound vibration "Ram" and the "Fire" element.

Asana Options
• Power Walk
• Jog
• Laughing Circle
• Spinal Twists
• Reversed Plank
• Boat
• Triangle
• Chair
• Warrior I
• Warrior II
• Bow
• Savasana with block on belly

Eating for This Chakra
Grains – pasta, bread, cereals, rice, flax seed, sunflower seed, etc.

Dairy – milk, cheese, yogurt.

Spices – ginger, mints (peppermint, spearmint, etc.), chamomile, turmeric, cumin, fennel.

Based on Chakra Three, Please Answer the Following Questions

When I truly look at myself, do I like what I see? Do I respect what I see? Do what others see define me?

_____
_____
_____
_____
_____
_____
_____
_____
_____
_____

When I am wrong, am I able to admit it?

_____
_____
_____
_____
_____
_____
_____
_____
_____
_____
_____

Do I understand the difference between "need" and "want?" When I use one, should I be using the other? How often does this happen?

_____
_____
_____
_____
_____
_____
_____
_____
_____

FOURTH CHAKRA — HEART CHAKRA — ANAHATA

I TAKE ACTION IN ACCORDANCE TO THE WISDOM OF MY HEART

Our fourth chakra is referred to as our heart chakra and governs our love, compassion and spirituality as it is the connection of the body and mind to the spirit. It serves to connect the three earthbound centers with that of the three spiritual centers. When this chakra is forgotten, a person may find themselves with an overwhelming feeling of sorrow for themselves. They may also experience a certain sense of indecisiveness or paranoia and may feel an unworthiness of love or a fear of getting hurt. This could translate to an inability to let go of feelings and things. If this chakra is put into balance, a person will see the good in people and things. They will unearth the gift of compassion, empathy, forgiveness and love for themselves and others.

The most prominent quality of this chakra is pure love. Oftentimes, we can mistake our feelings of love for those of lust or even greed. Pure unadulterated love gives without bias or reason. It is completely unconditional. When you relate to someone solely on a physical level, this isn't from the heart but from the mind. A mind does not love; it only wants. Once we've acquired what we seek, the grass will soon look greener elsewhere and we'll inevitably move on to our newest want.

When our hearts are open and pure, the Divine will manifest. But to truly open this chakra, we must first begin with a love for ourselves. If we do not have this, we cannot experience it from another. In loving ourselves, we create this feeling that is then shared with those around us. It will produce a balance.

Anahata Truths
• Sanskrit translation – unstruck sound
• Color – green
• Petals – 12
• Element – air
• Sound vibration, Bija Mantra – YAM
• Sense organ – skin, touch
• Develops – three to seven years
• Location – center of chest, heart center, heart
• Physical body – heart, lungs, respiratory and circulatory systems, arms, hands, thymus gland
• Physical imbalances – asthma, pneumonia, chronic bronchitis, upper back pain, shoulder pain, lung or breast cancer
• Emotional Imbalances – emotionally numb, feels empty,

Yoga Path
• Bhakti

Tools
• Oils – Orange Blossom, Rose, Bergamot, Jasmine, Lilac, Lavender, Rosemary
• Gems – Emerald, Green Jade, Rose Quartz, Boji Stone, Malachite, Green Tourmaline
• Incenses – Meadowsweet, Nag Champa, Orris Root

Tuning in With Breath
• Location
• Touch
• Contraction with Breath Retention

Tuning in With a Loving Peace Meditation
• Include the sound vibration "Yam" and the "Air" element.

Asana Options
• Bow
• Camel
• Hanuman
• Cow Face
• Cobra
• Fish
• Reclining Bound Angle

Eating for This Chakra
Leafy green vegetables – spinach, kale, swiss chard, dandelion greens, celery, etc.

Air vegetables – broccoli, cauliflower, cabbage, celery, squash, pumpkin, beans, peas, etc.

Grains – wheat, brown and white rice.

Liquids – green tea.

Spices – basil, sage, thyme, cilantro, parsley.

Based on Chakra Four, Please Answer the Following Questions

Do I understand the true meaning of compassion?

_____

_____

_____

_____

_____

_____

Do I understand the true meaning of forgiveness?

_____

_____

_____

_____

_____

_____

Do I understand the true meaning of intimacy?

_____

_____

_____

_____

_____

_____

Is there anything I have done that needs forgiveness? From whom? Has anything been done to me that needs forgiveness? For whom? Why haven't I yet?

_____

_____

_____

_____

_____

_____

FIFTH CHAKRA — THROAT CHAKRA — VISHUDDHA

BEFORE I SPEAK I PAUSE TO LISTEN CAREFULLY TO MY INNER TRUTH

Our fifth chakra is called the throat chakra and is the first of our chakras that focuses predominantly on the spiritual plane. It is this chakra that provides us the aptitude of our faith and understanding. It is the center of our will. It helps you realize that your life is your own. When it is not in balance, a person may discover an inability to express their thoughts in both word and deed. They may also experience moments of apprehension, weakness and anxiety. If it is unblocked, a person will enjoy the experience of being balanced or inspired and find their voice in situations where it wasn't there before. They will have the faith that the Universe will always provide. When vibrations of this center are high, you are content and see life from a higher level.

An important quality that we must cultivate for our spiritual growth is that of detachment. This isn't an unfeeling or cold detachment, but one that allows us to separate ourselves from the problems and obstacles we face each day. This chakra provides us with a sense of disentanglement, which lets us witness and observe life as it is. Consequently, we no longer are brought down by things we may understand as negative. We now see them as merely events on our path to the Divine. This shouldn't be confused with neglect of our own responsibility in what we say or do. But when we are faced with tremendous difficulty, we simply maintain a means by which we keep things in perspective. We choose to merely see.

Because this chakra is located in our throats, it governs our higher communication. It aids in our understanding of our inner truth and helps us through our voice and word to express it to that around us.

Vishuddha Truths
• Sanskrit translation – very pure
• Color – light bright turquoise
• Petals – 16
• Element – ether, space
• Sound vibration, Bija Mantra – HAM
• Sense organ – ear, hearing
• Develops – seven to twelve years
• Location – throat
• Physical body – mouth, tongue, throat, ears, eyes, shoulders, neck, thyroid and parathyroid gland
• Physical imbalances – speech issues, deafness
• Emotional imbalances – eating disorders

Yoga Path
• Mantra

Tools
• Oils – Bergamont, Chamomile, Eucalyptus, Sandalwood, Rea Tree, Peppermint
• Gems – Aquamarine, Turquoise, Amber, Amazonite, Lapis Lazuli, Amethyst
• Incenses – Myrrh Resin

Tuning in With Breath
• Location
• Touch
• Contraction with Breath Retention

Tuning in With a Purifying Meditation
• Include the sound vibration "Ham" and the "Ether, Space" element.

Asana Options
• Plow
• Fish
• Lion
• Neck Stretches
• Neck Rolls
• Reclining Neck Lifts

Eating for This Chakra
Tart or tangy fruits – lemon, lime, grapefruit, kiwi.

Tree fruit – apples, pears, plums, peaches, apricots, etc.

Liquids – water, fruit juice, herbal teas.

Spices – salt, lemongrass.

Based on Chakra Five, Please Answer the Following Questions

Is there an honesty and openness to how I express myself? If not, what is the reason?

_____
_____
_____
_____
_____
_____
_____
_____
_____

Do I listen to others? The universe? Am I heard by others? The universe?

_____
_____
_____
_____
_____
_____
_____
_____
_____
_____
_____

When in resonance, can I sense it? Do I use it?

_____
_____
_____
_____
_____
_____
_____
_____
_____
_____
_____

SIXTH CHAKRA — BROW CHAKRA — AJNA

I TRUST MY INTUITION TO GUIDE MY DECISIONS

Our sixth chakra is commonly known as our Third Eye or brow chakra and considered the perception center of our bodies. It is through this chakra that we are able to receive guidance and channel our Higher Selves. It is the energy center of traditional knowledge and important for developing a clear mind. When forgotten, we may find ourselves discouraged, insensitive, fearful of success and sometimes even egotistical. If kept open and in balance it will kindle our mystical side. It will connect us to our intuitive nature, influence our ability to see things others can't, and guide our capacity to see in our mind's eye our dreams or envision our future. We will understand we are our own master. It can even take us to an astral plane or to another time. But oftentimes these thoughts are so illogical that our minds cannot truly comprehend them and we are unable to make it real.

Those of us who wish to develop our sixth chakra can do so by uncovering our innate ability to look beyond the obvious. We need to free ourselves from all predetermined ideas of the things we encounter and observe them with brand new eyes. It is to see the truth and face it without fear. We often stunt the growth of this chakra through our inability to acknowledge our lack of knowledge, our need for help, or our necessity to learn different things. When we reject the legitimacy of unfamiliar ideas, we shut our minds off from this power. We become limited and look solely for the logical. It is then that we can no longer see.

When our Third Eye is open, we are no longer daunted by the obstacles that fall in our paths of life. We see them as opportunities to find alternative channels to achieve our purpose and rely on the intervention of the Divine. Things happen not by chance, but by design. Take time to calm our thoughts and focus on the here and now. Understand there is no one way to do, think or see. There are many means of living, none better or worse than the next.

Ajna Truths
• Sanskrit translation – command center
• Color – deep indigo blue
• Petals – 2
• Element – all elements
• Sound vibration, Bija Mantra – OM
• Sense organ – mind
• Develops – puberty
• Location – between brows, third eye
• Physical body – eyes, ears, nose, brow, base of skull, pineal gland
• Physical imbalances – voices inside head
• Emotional imbalances – vision problems, headaches, migraines, dizziness, poor memory, confusion, insomnia, acute sinusitis

Yoga Path
• Yantra

Tools
• Oils – Lemon, Juniper, Rosemary, Sandalwood, Lavender
• Gems – Lapis, Opal, Sapphire, Turquoise, Tiger's Eye, Amethyst
• Incenses – Frankincense, Sandalwood

Tuning in With Breath
• Location
• Touch
• Contraction with Breath Retention

Tuning in With a Intuition Meditation
• Include the sound vibration "Om" and "Light."

Asana Options
• Half Headstand
• Child's Pose
• Forward Fold
• Fish

Eating for This Chakra
Foods rich in chlorophyll – kale, wheatgrass, chlorella, sprouts, microgreens, seaweed.

Dark, bluish-colored fruits – red grapes, blueberries, blackberries, raspberries, etc.

Liquids – red wines and grape juice.

Spices – moringa, lavender, poppyseed, mugwort.

Based on Chakra Six, Please Answer the Following Questions

Do I receive guidance? Am I able to sense it and follow it?

_____
_____
_____
_____
_____
_____
_____

Do I have an internal vision of myself? What is it? Has it come to be?

_____
_____
_____
_____
_____
_____
_____

If not, do I understand how to fully realize it?

_____
_____
_____
_____
_____
_____
_____

Are there patterns in my life that I follow? Do they still fulfill a purpose?

_____
_____
_____
_____
_____
_____
_____

SEVENTH CHAKRA — CROWN CHAKRA — SAHASRARA

I GRACEFULLY ACCEPT WHAT THE UNIVERSE PRESENTS TO ME
TRUSTING THAT I AM EXACTLY WHERE I AM MEANT TO BE; ALL THINGS ARE CONNECTED

Our seventh chakra is commonly referred to as the Crown chakra and is said to connect us with the infinite or the Divine. Many believe that this is the location where the Soul enters at birth and exits at death. It is this chakra that joins together all the chakras with their individual qualities and allows for the inward flow of wisdom. Within this chakra, we will find our endowment of celestial consciousness. It serves as our connection to everything. If left neglected, a person may find themselves frustrated, disconnected or destructive. When put in balance, a person will find a certain sense of satisfaction in life, a connection to the world around them, and a productive nature to all that they do. They will unlock the doorway to both their unconscious and subconscious minds. They will experience their individual union with the Divine. It is here that our individual consciousness unites with the universal consciousness. We become enlightened.

As we awaken to the Divine, the limited becomes limitless. Our attachments lessen, our purposes become real and we radiate unconditional love and understanding. We uncover true empathy for all. Divine wisdom becomes ours.

Through a natural progression of work on the preceding chakras, our seventh chakra will mature and grow. We must come to terms with ourselves and rid judgment in our thoughts, words and deeds. We should nourish our spirituality. Find time for meditation or prayer. Listen to our instincts. Honor our God-given gifts. Live with purpose. Live with gratitude. Let the Divine animate your physical body.

Sahasrara Truths
- Sanskrit translation – infinite consciousness, thousand-petalled lotus
- Color – white, orchid, lavender, purple
- Petals – 1,000
- Element – all elements
- Sound vibration, Bija Mantra – OM – Silence
- Sense organ – conscious
- Develops – throughout life
- Location – top of head, beyond the senses
- Physical body – muscles, skeleton, skin, pituitary gland, CNS, cerebral cortex
- Physical imbalances – energetic disorders, chronic exhaustion or fatigue

Yoga Path
• Jnana

Tools
• Oils – Brahmi, Frankincense, Lavender, Hina Attar, Spikenard, Neroli
• Gems – Amethyst, Alexandrite, Crystal, Topaz, Citrine
• Incenses – Sandalwood, Sage, Cedar, Frankincense Resin, Myrrh Resin, Copal Resin, Juniper

Tuning in With Breath
• Location
• Touch
• Contraction with Breath Retention

Tuning in With a Consciousness Meditation
• Include the sound vibration "None" and "Thought."

Asana Options
• Effective Personal Practice
• Headstand
• Savasana

Eating for This Chakra
A pure, light vegetarian diet.

Based on Chakra Seven, Please Answer the Following Questions

Examine your beliefs about life, religion, and God. Then answer:

What are my actual beliefs in relation to life, religion and God?

_____
_____
_____
_____

Where do my beliefs stem from?

_____
_____
_____
_____

Who in my life shares these beliefs?

_____
_____
_____
_____

Do these beliefs affect the way I live my life?

_____
_____
_____
_____

Do I find contentment in these beliefs? How so?

_____
_____
_____
_____

Are these beliefs mine? Have they helped make me into the person I am today and will become tomorrow? Do my current beliefs shape the way I see others? Their words? Their actions? Are these views negative or positive?

_____
_____
_____
_____

Yoga Systems

I purposely list pranayama first in this section. Actual mention of asana in the Yoga Sutras is limited to very few passages, while breath and the levels of concentration, contemplation and pure meditation comprise a lot of the ancient text. Desikachar taught that pranayama is an excellent technique for entering a meditative state. On a physical body level, it is believed this allows for a connection of the sympathetic and parasympathetic nervous systems. Perhaps this opens up nerve pathways and release of hormones that bring an enhanced sense of calm to the individual. Chanting adds depth to this practice. The vibrational frequency resonates within the jawbone and skull, possibly acting as a tuning fork for our brain frequency.

I always say that once we disconnect from focus on the breath, it's not yoga. Many yogis consider the diaphragm to be the spiritual muscle – bringing our first and last breath in this lifetime. Ultimately, as one practices yoga faithfully, we develop a spiritual connection. Savasana, also called corpse pose, is at the end of every session because we practice the subtle energy associated with the Soul passing from the physical plane. Good yoga teachers allow sufficient time for Savasana as we settle into our own being through this relaxation. Ask your yoga teacher to practice 10 minutes of Savasana for every hour of yoga. Bring Savasana into your personal practice as well. You will reap calming benefits from doing so.

Recently, it seems that people are more interested in the "style" of yoga than the benefits of yoga. The biggest question I get is, "What style do you teach?" But I do note an emerging trend among the students attracted to my teacher training. What they practice isn't working for them. The style is less meaningful after a while. They are getting hurt or notice yoga instructions that are not safe. It's too fast to relax. The context is missing and so are the benefits, other than a good stretchy workout. They seek another way – an accommodating and inclusive way to practice yoga with intention and focus on what benefits this practice can bring to them.

The human body was designed to move. From the double helix design of our DNA to the unique balanced tension design of our spine, we are made up of potential energy that requires movement to stay in tune, in balance. When we don't move, we get out of balance. Our bodies start to accept the position we are in and grows tissue to be in that position. Limited cycles of movement are introduced and we feel pain when we call upon our bodies to move in a new direction.

I always say, "If it's not about the breath and the spine, it's not yoga." Asana means "comfortable seat." It is the part of yoga as a whole that most people in the West think of when they hear the word "yoga." But in fact, the purpose of asana is to prepare the body for meditation, which is very important.

The benefits of asana are many and they include –
• Keeps the spinal column supple.
• Settles the mind.
• Settles the senses.
• Settles prana and energy.

When practicing asana, here are a few basic concepts to keep in mind –
• All yoga postures originate from the spine.
• Always move the spine six ways.
• Your breath is your teacher and your guide. It will take you to your limit.
• Always find a neutral spine in each posture and start from there.
• The best way to align the body is with gravity. Work with the structure of the body, not against it.
• Always do a general warm-up – bringing blood flow to the muscles, synovial fluid flow to the joints, length and space to connective tissues.
• Work your way out to the limbs.
• Use both static and dynamic postures in each practice.
• Always do counter-poses with a neutral posture in between.
• Practice in a way to touch all layers of the body – physical, energetic, mental, intellectual, spiritual.
• Set long-term and short-term goals for yourself and your students.
• Practice with your whole mind, body and Soul.
• Practice, practice, practice.
• Consistency of practice will lead to consistency in results.

Like the systems of a clock – a yoga practice must include breathing, moving, meditation. Meditation has been proven to build calmer aspects to the brain. Allowing the brain to turn off, the mind to relax a bit, involves practice and patience. Don't worry – it's all good. For when you can focus on one thing, you train your mind to turn off the senses. It relaxes. Just a few minutes are required each day. More can be better though. The lovely thing about meditation is that it does not involve leggings, props or the right setting. Meditation can be practiced most anywhere (okay, Times Square does present its challenges).

As one reaches deeper levels of meditation, great insights can be received. We just have to slow down, calm down and understand that this yoga state is the place to which we were born and will revisit again one day. Why not practice going there every day?

PRANAYAMA

Breath practice, or pranayama, is the fourth limb of the eight limbs of yoga. The easiest method of looking at pranayama is through translation. The word itself can be broken out into two separate halves. The first is that of prana, which we know signifies vital energy. The second is that of yama, denoting the act of control. Together the two halves translate as control of vital energy. Since vital energy is said to enter the body through our breath, pranayama is the practice of controlling one's breath.

The actual practice of pranayama is believed to begin with a shift in the practitioner's awareness, moving from the outside world in which we all reside to that of the inner essence. You can think of it as moving your consciousness from the body to the mind, which allows you to move closer to the Self. It's the vehicle used to harness the breath in order to circulate vital energy throughout the body and thereby find peace within.

If you were to strictly follow Patanjali's teachings, you would understand that you must first learn to control the body before moving into the practice of pranayama. Today this is rarely done. Most yoga instructors expose their students to breathing exercises in the first few sessions together. Does this mean that people are being taught an incorrect approach to yoga? Not necessarily, since even Patanjali himself didn't consider the perfection of posture a prerequisite of practice. To truly apply pranayama to yoga, you must be able to sit in steadiness and ease.

Natural Breath, the Way God Intended
Natural breath is one of the common breathing practices of pranayama. Often referred to as abdominal breath or diaphragmatic breathing, it's the act of breathing deeply into the lungs by fully engaging the diaphragm. It's essentially belly breathing since you extend the lower abdomen to deepen your breath. The act of natural breath starts with prolonged inhalation through the nostrils and moves to a delayed retention of breath before deeply exhaling through the mouth. Each exhalation is followed with another delayed retention prior to your next inhalation.

Breath Journal
Please record the number of breaths you take in a minute, for several days, and at different times of the day.

Date _____ Time of Day _____ # of Breaths per minute _____

Date _____ Time of Day _____ # of Breaths per minute _____

Date _____ Time of Day _____ # of Breaths per minute _____

Date _____ Time of Day _____ # of Breaths per minute _____

Date _____ Time of Day _____ # of Breaths per minute _____

Date _____ Time of Day _____ # of Breaths per minute _____

Date _____ Time of Day _____ # of Breaths per minute _____

Date _____ Time of Day _____ # of Breaths per minute _____

Date _____ Time of Day _____ # of Breaths per minute _____

The Bellos Breath – Bhastrika Pranayama
- week 1 - 10 rounds
- week 2 - 15 rounds
- week 3 - 20 rounds
- week 4 - 25 rounds
- week 5 - 30 rounds
- do no more than five minutes at a time

Skull Shining Breath – Kapalabhati Pranayama
- week 1 - 10 rounds
- week 2 - 15 rounds
- week 3 - 20 rounds
- week 4 - 25 rounds
- week 5 - 30 rounds
- do no more than five minutes at a time

Alternate Nostril Breath – Nadi Shodhana Pranayama
- week 1 - 10 rounds
- week 2 - 20 rounds
- week 3 - 30 rounds
- week 4 - 40 rounds
- week 5 - 50 rounds
- do no more than ten minutes at a time

Humming Bee Breath – Bhramari Pranayama
- week 1 - 10 rounds
- week 2 - 20 rounds
- week 3 - 30 rounds
- week 4 - 40 rounds
- week 5 - 50 rounds
- do no more than ten minutes at a time

Victorious Breath – Ujjayi Pranayama
- week 1 - 10 rounds
- week 2 - 20 rounds
- week 3 - 30 rounds
- week 4 - 40 rounds
- week 5 - 50 rounds
- can practice all the time

Fire Essence Breath – Agnisar Pranayama
- week 1 - 5 breaths
- week 2 - 10 breaths
- week 3 - 15 breaths
- week 4 - 20 breaths
- week 5 - 25 breaths
- do no more than five minutes at a time

ASANA

NO ONE IS WISE BY BIRTH. WISDOM RESULTS FROM ONES OWN EFFORTS ~ KRISHNAMACHARYA

Build Your Own Mini Sequence for Yourself or a Real Person You Know

• Who is this sequence for?

• What is your objective?

• What do you hope to accomplish?

• How long is this sequence?

• What is your approach?

• What is the reason for each posture you chose?

• Does the purpose of each posture fit with your clients needs? Lifestyle?

• Will your client grow in their life's purpose with this sequence?

• Do you need any props?

Asana Awarness

In order to teach a pose properly, you must be able to teach that pose for 32 minutes and you must be able stay in that pose for 10 minutes. Take a deep breath and relax. This is a process in development. Layer by layer. Talking point by talking point.

Really Real Yoga

Always be mindful of your heart-mind. Sankalpa is a impression formed in the heart-mind, often experienced during the practice of yoga nidra, although experiencing Sankalpa is possible anytime.

Standing Postures

Cautions – Standing Postures Should be Avoided When
• Students are experiencing the first few days of their menstrual cycle.
• Students are in the first three months of pregnancy, or completely if a students is experiencing a problem pregnancy.
• Students have heart conditions, high or low blood pressure.
• Students have a back injury or tenderness in the low back.
• Students have varicose veins.
• Students have diarrhea or similar symptoms.
• Students have fractures and compressed nerves.

Benefits – Standing Postures Should be Practiced to
• Build strength and balance throughout the body.
• Work the major muscle groups of the body.
• Help develop inner focus.
• Invigorate the mind.
• Bring vitality to the Self.
• Stimulate digestion and elimination.
• Regulate kidney function.
• Help with constipation.
• Improve circulation.
• Increase lung capacity.
• Strengthen the muscles of heart and tone cardiovascular system.
• Develop strength in the lower body, shoulders and neck.
• Tone buttocks muscles and reduces fat in hips and waist area.
• Help increase flexibility of the pelvis, lower back and spine.
• Teach alignment through a firm foundation.
• Strengthen the spine.
• Help improve comfort during menstruation when practiced everyday.

Seated Postures

Cautions – Seated Postures Should be Avoided When
• Students have injured, tender, or tight hips.
• Students have back, knee, or ankle injuries.
• Students have asthma.
• Students have difficulty getting up from and down to the floor.

Benefits – Seated Postures Should be Practiced to
• Soothe nerves.
• Improve circulation.
• Bring calmness.
• Eliminate fatigue.
• Increase blood flow throughout body.
• Refreshe the brain.
• Regulate blood pressure.
• Help facilitate restful night's sleep.
• Strengthen the muscles of chest.
• Remove tension in the diaphragm and throat, helping to ease the breath.
• Relieve backaches.
• Ease stiffness of the joints.
• Help improve comfort during menstrual cycles.
• Tone abdominal muscles and organs.
• Tone leg muscles and open hips and groin.
• Bring peace of mind from a steady spine.

Inversions

Cautions – Inversions Should Be Avoided When
• Students are experiencing the heaviest days of the menstrual cycle.
• Students are pregnant, especially students very late in their pregnancy.
• Students have hand, wrist, elbow, back, neck, or shoulder injuries.
• Students have heart conditions, high or low blood pressure.
• Students are experiencing a headache or migrane.
• Students have detached retina, glaucoma, general eye problems.
• Students have poor hearing, vertigo, or general dizziness.
• Students have diarrhea or similar symptoms.
• Students have acid reflux or gastroesophageal reflux (GERD).
• Students are diabetic.

Benefits – Inversions Should be Practiced to
• Bring fresh blood to the head and heart.
• Improve circulation.
• Bring mental strength.
• Reverse the flow of lymph fluid.
• Help treat the common cold and other throat ailments.
• Stimulate brain function and rejuvenate the body.
• Relieve fatigue and boosts energy levels.
• Tone and strengthens internal organs.
• Refresh tired legs.
• Strengthen the muscles of the neck.

Twisting and Extending Postures

Cautions – Twists and Extending Postures Should Be Avoided When
• Students have back injuries.
• Students have difficulty balancing.
• Students have poor eye sight.
• Students are suffering from diarrhea or similar symptoms.
• Students have high or low blood pressure.
• Students are pregnant.

Benefits – Twisting and Extending Postures Should be Practiced to
• Balance and energize the body.
• Improve blood flow to the spinal nerves.
• Increase energy levels.
• Tone and stimulate the pelvic and abdominal organs.
• Help with digestion.
• Relieve constipation.
• Help improve comfort during menstrual cycles.
• Help keep the spine and shoulders supple.
• Teache the importance of a healthy spine and inner body.
• Relieve pain in the neck, shoulders and back.
• Increase flexibility in spine and hips.
• Improve suppleness of the diaphragm.
• Relieve spinal, hip and groin disorders.
• Reduce fat around the waistline.

Forward Folding Postures

Cautions – Forward Folds Should Be Avoided When
• Students have a back injury or tenderness in the low back.
• Students have heart conditions, high or low blood pressure.
• Students have difficulty balancing.
• Students suffer from blocked sinuses or have difficulty breathing
• Students have poor eye sight.
• Students have diarrhea or similar symptoms.
• Students who are pregnant, especially students very late in their pregnancy.

Benefits – Forward Folding Postures Should be Practiced to
• Stretch the lower back and lengthen hamstrings.
• Aid in digestion.
• Strengthen the back and legs.
• Relieve fatigue.
• Soothe the nervous system.
• Rejuvenate the body.
• Refresh the mind.
• Restore energy (if incorporated at the end of a practice).
• Help improve comfort during menstrual cycles.
• Reduce cardiac disorders.
• Bring one into the highest state of consciousness.
• Bring one into a state of deep relaxation.
• Regulate the breath.
• Bring calmness to the body.

Backbending Postures

Cautions – Backbending Postures Should Be Avoided When
• Students have heart conditions, high or low blood pressure.
• Students are experiencing the first few days of their menstrual cycle.
• Students who are pregnant, especially students very late in their pregnancy.
• Students with hand wrist, elbow, or arm injuries.
• Students with back injuries or students with tender low back.
• Students with generally weak bodies, especially if weak in around the torso and shoulders.
• Students who are especially tight in the thoracic spine.

Benefits – Backbending Postures Should be Practiced to
• Bring a state of liveliness to the body and mind.
• Open and energize the body.
• Develop courage.
• Help alleviate depression headaches, hypertension, and nervous exhaustion.
• Open the chest.
• Increase lung capacity.
• Improve circulation to the organs.
• Stimulate the nervous system, increasing the body's ability to bear stress.
• Strengthen arms, shoulders, back, hips and legs.
• Increase flexibility of the spine.
• Improve posture.
• Help improve comfort during menstrual cycles.
• Stretch organs, allowing them to function more effectively.

Bound Angle - Baddha Konasana - (bha-dah cone-ahs-anna)
       (baddha = bound) (kona = angle)

Benefits

• Consistent practice of this pose until late into pregnancy is said to help ease childbirth.

• Stimulates abdominal organs, ovaries and prostate gland, bladder, and kidneys - how?

• Traditional texts say that Baddha Konasana destroys disease and gets rid of fatigue.

• Therapeutic for flat feet, high blood pressure, infertility, and asthma - why?

• Helps relieve mild depression, anxiety, and fatigue - cautions?

• Stimulates the heart and improves general circulation - how?

• Stretches the inner thighs, groins, and knees - cautions?

• Soothes menstrual discomfort and sciatica - cautions?

• Helps relieve the symptoms of menopause - why?

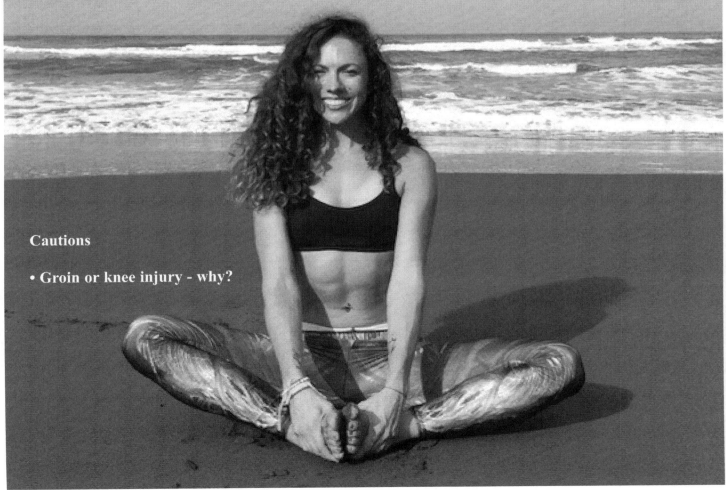

Cautions

• Groin or knee injury - why?

Anatomical Sheath – Annamaya Kosha – Physical Layer – Muscles and bones, then organs.
Muscles and Bones

_____

_____

Organs

_____

_____

List physical direction cues in order. Reminder, "all yoga postures originate from the spine."
Would you teach this posture from the ground up or the spine out?

_____

_____

Marianne's "-3 -2 -1 0 1 2 3"
List 3 ways to reduce this posture   List 3 ways to enhance this posture

_____   _____

_____   _____

List 3 Preparatory Postures   List 3 Subsequent Postures

_____   _____

_____   _____

Life Force Sheath – Pranamaya Kosha – Altered states of energetics through breath regulation.
How does your breath flow in this pose? Where do you get stuck? Where can you direct the breath?

_____

_____

Mental Sheath – Manomaya Kosha – Our fluctuating mental and emotional layer.
How can this posture calm the fluctuations of the mind and emotions? Does the physical body interfere?

_____

_____

Next Steps After Training, Pause and Reflect on –

Intellectual Sheath – Vijnanamaya Kosha – Self-study beyond thought, pure witness.
Have you ever experienced this place of pure space in this posture?

Bliss Sheath – Anandamaya Kosha – Love, Joy, Peace, Freedom
How does this posture help you move closer to the spiritualness of yoga?

Use the space below to draw this posture.

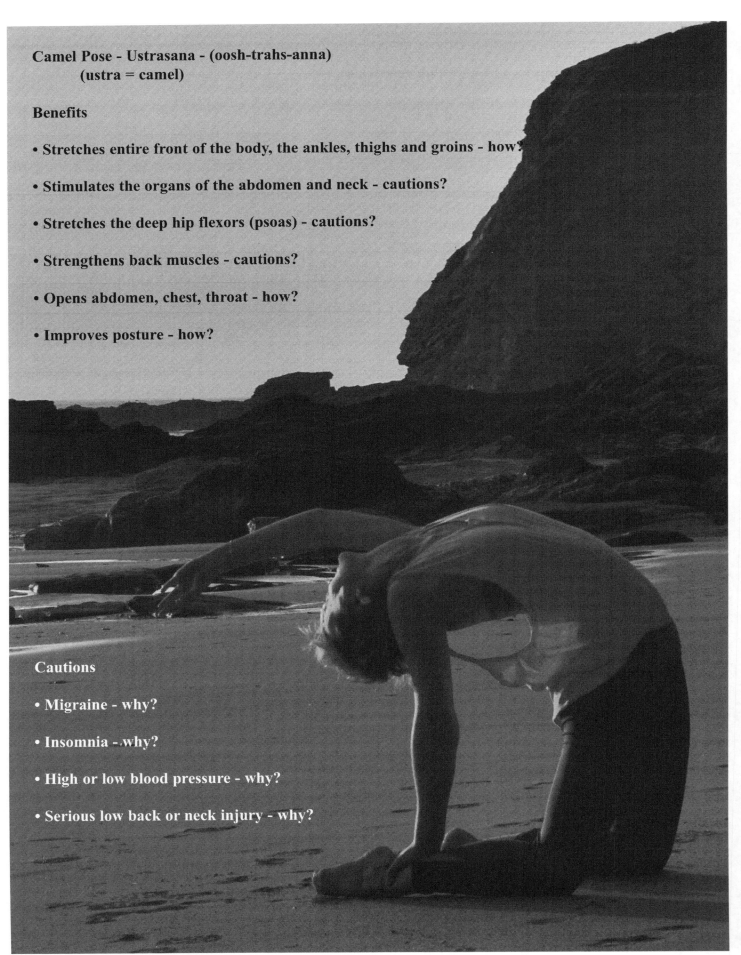

Camel Pose - Ustrasana - (oosh-trahs-anna)
     (ustra = camel)

Benefits

• Stretches entire front of the body, the ankles, thighs and groins - how?

• Stimulates the organs of the abdomen and neck - cautions?

• Stretches the deep hip flexors (psoas) - cautions?

• Strengthens back muscles - cautions?

• Opens abdomen, chest, throat - how?

• Improves posture - how?

Cautions

• Migraine - why?

• Insomnia - why?

• High or low blood pressure - why?

• Serious low back or neck injury - why?

Anatomical Sheath – Annamaya Kosha – Physical Layer – Muscles and bones, then organs.
Muscles and Bones
_____
_____
_____

Organs
_____
_____
_____

List physical direction cues in order. Reminder, "all yoga postures originate from the spine."
Would you teach this posture from the ground up or the spine out?
_____
_____
_____

Marianne's "-3 -2 -1 0 1 2 3"

List 3 ways to reduce this posture   List 3 ways to enhance this posture
_____   _____
_____   _____
_____   _____

List 3 Preparatory Postures   List 3 Subsequent Postures
_____   _____
_____   _____
_____   _____

Life Force Sheath – Pranamaya Kosha – Altered states of energetics through breath regulation.
How does your breath flow in this pose? Where do you get stuck? Where can you direct the breath?
_____
_____
_____

Mental Sheath – Manomaya Kosha – Our fluctuating mental and emotional layer.
How can this posture calm the fluctuations of the mind and emotions? Does the physical body interfere?
_____
_____
_____

Next Steps After Training, Pause and Reflect on –

Intellectual Sheath – Vijnanamaya Kosha – Self-study beyond thought, pure witness.
Have you ever experienced this place of pure space in this posture?

Bliss Sheath – Anandamaya Kosha – Love, Joy, Peace, Freedom
How does this posture help you move closer to the spiritualness of yoga?

Use the space below to draw this posture.

Lord of the Dance Pose - Natarajasana - (not-ah-raj-ahs-anna)
        (nata = dancer) (raja = king)

Benefits

• **Stretches shoulders, chest, abdomen, thighs and groins - how?**

• **Strengthens back, abdomen, legs and ankles - how?**

• **Improves balance and focus - how?**

Cautions

• **High or low blood pressure - why?**

• **Low back problems - why?**

• **Diarrhea - why?**

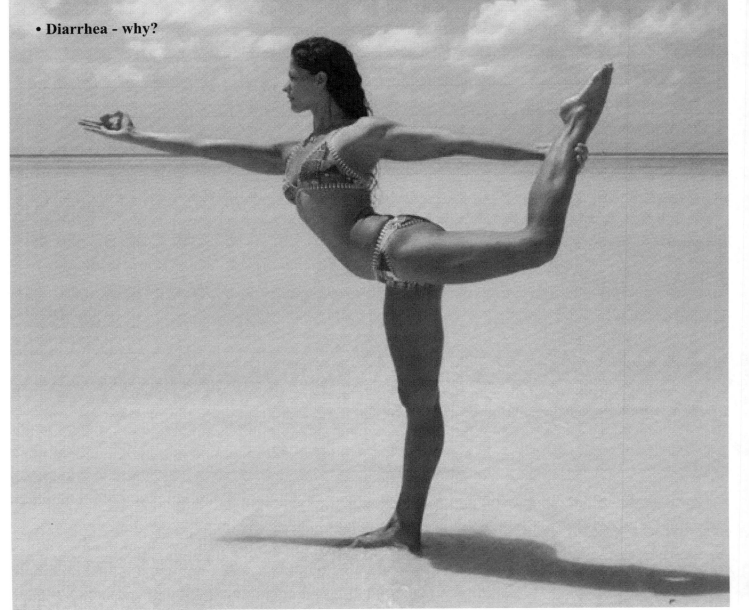

Anatomical Sheath – Annamaya Kosha – Physical Layer – Muscles and bones, then organs.
Muscles and Bones

_____

_____

Organs

_____

_____

List physical direction cues in order. Reminder, "all yoga postures originate from the spine."
Would you teach this posture from the ground up or the spine out?

_____

_____

Marianne's "-3 -2 -1 0 1 2 3"
List 3 ways to reduce this posture   List 3 ways to enhance this posture

_____   _____

_____   _____

List 3 Preparatory Postures   List 3 Subsequent Postures

_____   _____

_____   _____

Life Force Sheath – Pranamaya Kosha – Altered states of energetics through breath regulation.
How does your breath flow in this pose? Where do you get stuck? Where can you direct the breath?

_____

_____

Mental Sheath – Manomaya Kosha – Our fluctuating mental and emotional layer.
How can this posture calm the fluctuations of the mind and emotions? Does the physical body interfere?

_____

_____

Next Steps After Training, Pause and Reflect on –

Intellectual Sheath – Vijnanamaya Kosha – Self-study beyond thought, pure witness.
Have you ever experienced this place of pure space in this posture?

Bliss Sheath – Anandamaya Kosha – Love, Joy, Peace, Freedom
How does this posture help you move closer to the spiritualness of yoga?

Use the space below to draw this posture.

Downward Facing Dog - Adho Mukha Svanasana - (ah-doh moo-kah shvah-nahs-anna)
(adho = downward) (mukha = face) (svana = dog)

Benefits

• Therapeutic for high blood pressure, asthma, flat feet, sciatica, sinusitis - how?

• Stretches the shoulders, hamstrings, calves, arches, and hands - cautions?

• Relieves menstrual discomfort when done with head supported - how?

• Calms the brain and helps relieve stress and mild depression - how?

• Relieves headache, insomnia, back pain, and fatigue - how?

• Helps relieve the symptoms of menopause - how?

• Strengthens the arms and legs - cautions?

• Helps prevent osteoporosis - how?

• Energizes the body - how?

• Improves digestion - how?

Cautions

• Diarrhea - why?

• Headache - why?

• Carpal tunnel syndrome - why?

• High or low blood pressure - why?

• Pregnancy, do not do this pose in third trimester - why?

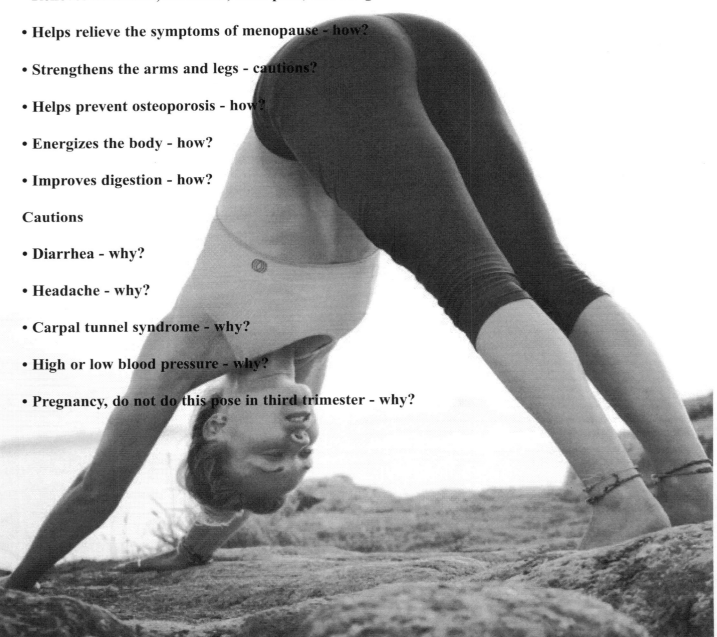

Anatomical Sheath – Annamaya Kosha – Physical Layer – Muscles and bones, then organs.
Muscles and Bones
_____
_____

Organs
_____
_____

List physical direction cues in order. Reminder, "all yoga postures originate from the spine."
Would you teach this posture from the ground up or the spine out?
_____
_____

Marianne's "-3 -2 -1 0 1 2 3"
List 3 ways to reduce this posture   List 3 ways to enhance this posture
_____   _____
_____   _____

List 3 Preparatory Postures   List 3 Subsequent Postures
_____   _____
_____   _____

Life Force Sheath – Pranamaya Kosha – Altered states of energetics through breath regulation.
How does your breath flow in this pose? Where do you get stuck? Where can you direct the breath?
_____
_____

Mental Sheath – Manomaya Kosha – Our fluctuating mental and emotional layer.
How can this posture calm the fluctuations of the mind and emotions? Does the physical body interfere?
_____
_____

Next Steps After Training, Pause and Reflect on –

Intellectual Sheath – Vijnanamaya Kosha – Self-study beyond thought, pure witness.
Have you ever experienced this place of pure space in this posture?

Bliss Sheath – Anandamaya Kosha – Love, Joy, Peace, Freedom
How does this posture help you move closer to the spiritualness of yoga?

Use the space below to draw this posture. ✍️🖋️🖋️🖋️

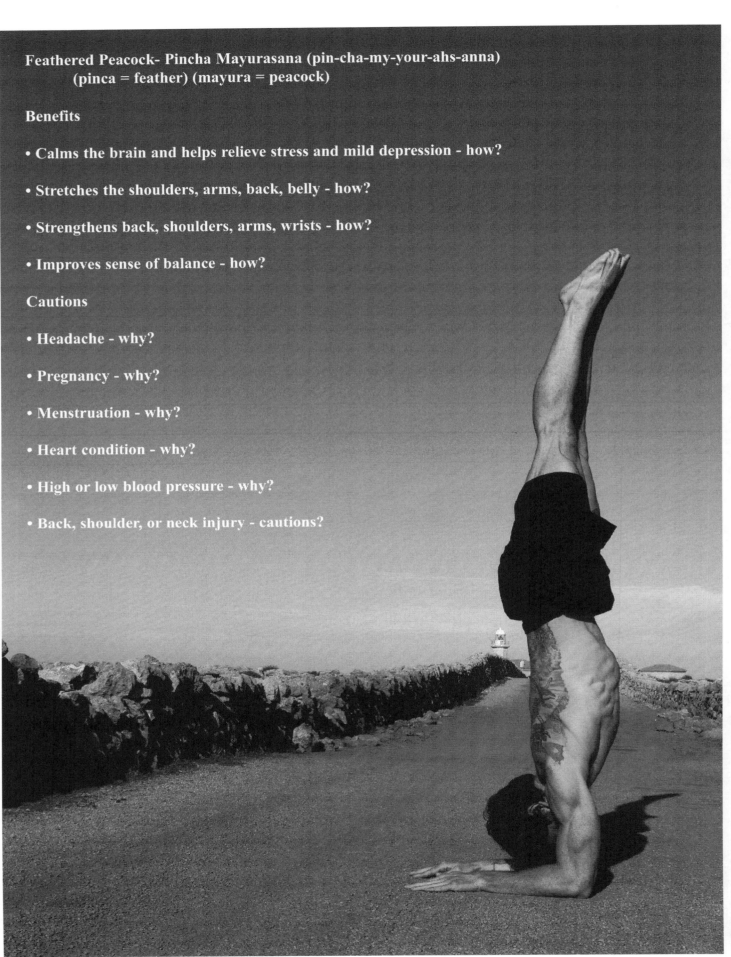

Feathered Peacock- Pincha Mayurasana (pin-cha-my-your-ahs-anna)
        (pinca = feather) (mayura = peacock)

Benefits

• Calms the brain and helps relieve stress and mild depression - how?

• Stretches the shoulders, arms, back, belly - how?

• Strengthens back, shoulders, arms, wrists - how?

• Improves sense of balance - how?

Cautions

• Headache - why?

• Pregnancy - why?

• Menstruation - why?

• Heart condition - why?

• High or low blood pressure - why?

• Back, shoulder, or neck injury - cautions?

Anatomical Sheath – Annamaya Kosha – Physical Layer – Muscles and bones, then organs.
Muscles and Bones
_____
_____
_____

Organs
_____
_____

List physical direction cues in order. Reminder, "all yoga postures originate from the spine."
Would you teach this posture from the ground up or the spine out?
_____
_____
_____

Marianne's "-3 -2 -1 0 1 2 3"
List 3 ways to reduce this posture

List 3 ways to enhance this posture

_____
_____

_____
_____

List 3 Preparatory Postures

List 3 Subsequent Postures

_____
_____

_____
_____

Life Force Sheath – Pranamaya Kosha – Altered states of energetics through breath regulation.
How does your breath flow in this pose? Where do you get stuck? Where can you direct the breath?
_____
_____
_____

Mental Sheath – Manomaya Kosha – Our fluctuating mental and emotional layer.
How can this posture calm the fluctuations of the mind and emotions? Does the physical body interfere?
_____
_____
_____

Next Steps After Training, Pause and Reflect on –

Intellectual Sheath – Vijnanamaya Kosha – Self-study beyond thought, pure witness.
Have you ever experienced this place of pure space in this posture?

Bliss Sheath – Anandamaya Kosha – Love, Joy, Peace, Freedom
How does this posture help you move closer to the spiritualness of yoga?

Use the space below to draw this posture. ✍✎✎✎

Handstand - Adho Mukha Vrksasana (ah-doh-moo-kah-vriks-shahs-anna)
(adho = downward) (mukha = face) (vrksa = tree)

Benefits

• Calms the brain and helps relieve stress and mild depression - how?

• Strengthens shoulders, arms, wrists - how?

• Improves sense of balance - how?

• Stretches the belly - how?

Cautions

• Headache - why?

• Pregnancy - why?

• Menstruation - why?

• Heart condition - why?

• High or low blood pressure - why?

Anatomical Sheath – Annamaya Kosha – Physical Layer – Muscles and bones, then organs.
Muscles and Bones

_____
_____

Organs

_____
_____

List physical direction cues in order. Reminder, "all yoga postures originate from the spine."
Would you teach this posture from the ground up or the spine out?

_____
_____

Marianne's "-3 -2 -1 0 1 2 3"
List 3 ways to reduce this posture   List 3 ways to enhance this posture

_____   _____
_____   _____

List 3 Preparatory Postures   List 3 Subsequent Postures

_____   _____
_____   _____
_____   _____

Life Force Sheath – Pranamaya Kosha – Altered states of energetics through breath regulation.
How does your breath flow in this pose? Where do you get stuck? Where can you direct the breath?

_____
_____
_____

Mental Sheath – Manomaya Kosha – Our fluctuating mental and emotional layer.
How can this posture calm the fluctuations of the mind and emotions? Does the physical body interfere?

_____
_____
_____

Next Steps After Training, Pause and Reflect on –

Intellectual Sheath – Vijnanamaya Kosha – Self-study beyond thought, pure witness.
Have you ever experienced this place of pure space in this posture?

Bliss Sheath – Anandamaya Kosha – Love, Joy, Peace, Freedom
How does this posture help you move closer to the spiritualness of yoga?

Use the space below to draw this posture.

Supported Headstand - Salamba Sirsasana - (sah-lom-bah shear-shahs-anna)
(sa = with) (alamba = support) (sirsa = head)

Benefits

• Calms the brain and helps relieve stress and mild depression - how?

• Therapeutic for asthma, infertility, insomnia, and sinusitis - why?

• Strengthens the arms, legs, spine and lungs - how?

• Helps relieve the symptoms of menopause - how?

• Stimulates the pituitary and pineal glands - how?

• Tones the abdominal organs - how?

• Improves digestion - how?

Cautions

• Headache - why?

• Menstruation - why?

• Heart condition - why?

• Back or neck injury - why?

• High or low blood pressure - why?

• Do not continue to practice late into pregnancy.

Anatomical Sheath – Annamaya Kosha – Physical Layer – Muscles and bones, then organs.

Muscles and Bones
_____

_____

Organs
_____

_____

List physical direction cues in order. Reminder, "all yoga postures originate from the spine."
Would you teach this posture from the ground up or the spine out?
_____

_____

Marianne's "-3 -2 -1 0 1 2 3"

List 3 ways to reduce this posture

_____

_____

List 3 Preparatory Postures

_____

_____

List 3 ways to enhance this posture

_____

_____

List 3 Subsequent Postures

_____

_____

Life Force Sheath – Pranamaya Kosha – Altered states of energetics through breath regulation.
How does your breath flow in this pose? Where do you get stuck? Where can you direct the breath?
_____

_____

Mental Sheath – Manomaya Kosha – Our fluctuating mental and emotional layer.
How can this posture calm the fluctuations of the mind and emotions? Does the physical body interfere?
_____

_____

Next Steps After Training, Pause and Reflect on –

Intellectual Sheath – Vijnanamaya Kosha – Self-study beyond thought, pure witness.
Have you ever experienced this place of pure space in this posture?

Bliss Sheath – Anandamaya Kosha – Love, Joy, Peace, Freedom
How does this posture help you move closer to the spiritualness of yoga?

Use the space below to draw this posture.

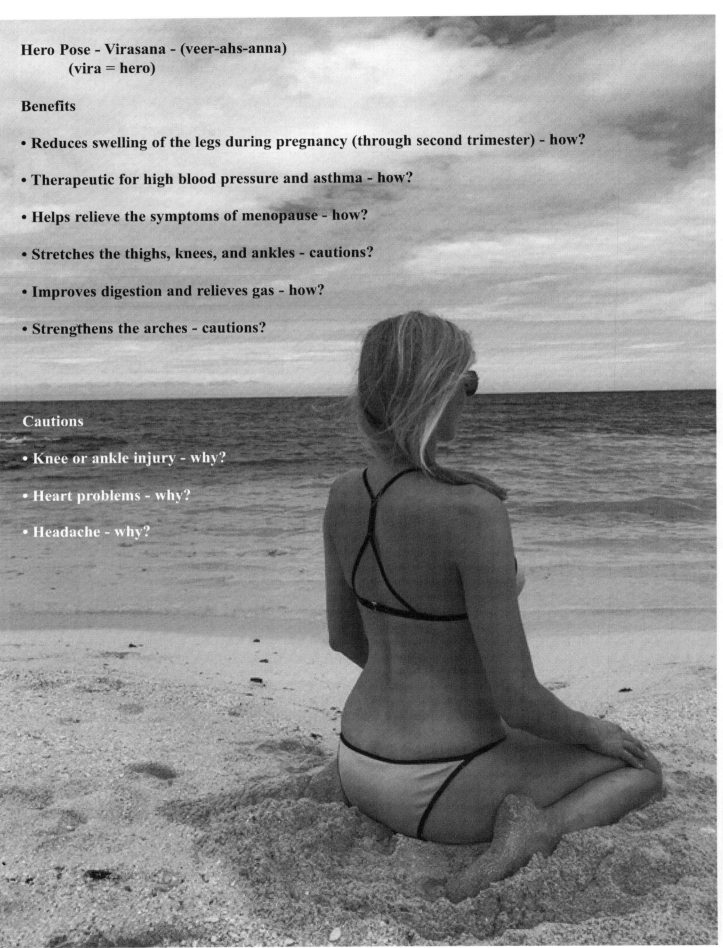

Hero Pose - Virasana - (veer-ahs-anna)
        (vira = hero)

Benefits

• **Reduces swelling of the legs during pregnancy (through second trimester) - how?**

• **Therapeutic for high blood pressure and asthma - how?**

• **Helps relieve the symptoms of menopause - how?**

• **Stretches the thighs, knees, and ankles - cautions?**

• **Improves digestion and relieves gas - how?**

• **Strengthens the arches - cautions?**

Cautions

• **Knee or ankle injury - why?**

• **Heart problems - why?**

• **Headache - why?**

Anatomical Sheath – Annamaya Kosha – Physical Layer – Muscles and bones, then organs.
Muscles and Bones

_____

_____

Organs

_____

_____

List physical direction cues in order. Reminder, "all yoga postures originate from the spine."
Would you teach this posture from the ground up or the spine out?

_____

_____

Marianne's "-3 -2 -1 0 1 2 3"
List 3 ways to reduce this posture   List 3 ways to enhance this posture

_____   _____

_____   _____

_____   _____

List 3 Preparatory Postures   List 3 Subsequent Postures

_____   _____

_____   _____

_____   _____

Life Force Sheath – Pranamaya Kosha – Altered states of energetics through breath regulation.
How does your breath flow in this pose? Where do you get stuck? Where can you direct the breath?

_____

_____

_____

Mental Sheath – Manomaya Kosha – Our fluctuating mental and emotional layer.
How can this posture calm the fluctuations of the mind and emotions? Does the physical body interfere?

_____

_____

_____

Next Steps After Training, Pause and Reflect on –

Intellectual Sheath – Vijnanamaya Kosha – Self-study beyond thought, pure witness.
Have you ever experienced this place of pure space in this posture?

Bliss Sheath – Anandamaya Kosha – Love, Joy, Peace, Freedom
How does this posture help you move closer to the spiritualness of yoga?

Use the space below to draw this posture. ✍🖊🖊🖊

Intense Side Stretch - Parsvottanasana - (parsh-voh-tahn-ahs-anna)
       (parsva = side, flank) (ut = intense) (tan = to extend)

Benefits

• Stretches spine, shoulders and wrists (in the full pose), hips, and hamstrings - cautions?

• Stimulates the abdominal organs, improving digestion - cautions?

• Calms the brain, improving posture and sense of balance - how?

• Strengthens the legs - cautions?

Cautions

• Back injury - why?

• High or low blood pressure - why?

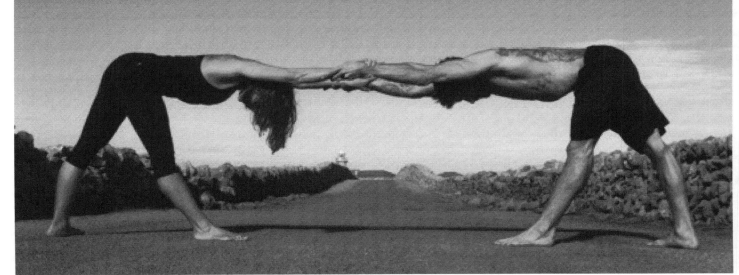

Anatomical Sheath – Annamaya Kosha – Physical Layer – Muscles and bones, then organs.
Muscles and Bones

_____

_____

Organs

_____

_____

List physical direction cues in order. Reminder, "all yoga postures originate from the spine."
Would you teach this posture from the ground up or the spine out?

_____

_____

Marianne's "-3 -2 -1 0 1 2 3"
List 3 ways to reduce this posture   List 3 ways to enhance this posture

_____   _____

_____   _____

List 3 Preparatory Postures   List 3 Subsequent Postures

_____   _____

_____   _____

Life Force Sheath – Pranamaya Kosha – Altered states of energetics through breath regulation.
How does your breath flow in this pose? Where do you get stuck? Where can you direct the breath?

_____

_____

Mental Sheath – Manomaya Kosha – Our fluctuating mental and emotional layer.
How can this posture calm the fluctuations of the mind and emotions? Does the physical body interfere?

_____

_____

Next Steps After Training, Pause and Reflect on –

Intellectual Sheath – Vijnanamaya Kosha – Self-study beyond thought, pure witness.
Have you ever experienced this place of pure space in this posture?

Bliss Sheath – Anandamaya Kosha – Love, Joy, Peace, Freedom
How does this posture help you move closer to the spiritualness of yoga?

Use the space below to draw this posture.

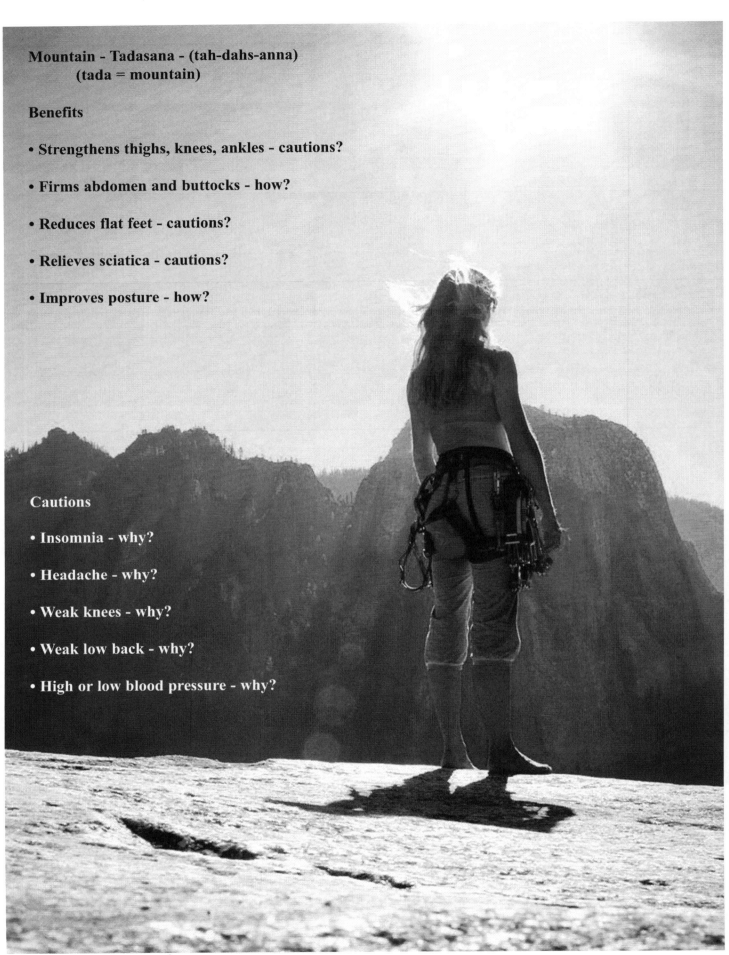

Mountain - Tadasana - (tah-dahs-anna)
       (tada = mountain)

Benefits

• **Strengthens thighs, knees, ankles - cautions?**

• **Firms abdomen and buttocks - how?**

• **Reduces flat feet - cautions?**

• **Relieves sciatica - cautions?**

• **Improves posture - how?**

Cautions

• **Insomnia - why?**

• **Headache - why?**

• **Weak knees - why?**

• **Weak low back - why?**

• **High or low blood pressure - why?**

Anatomical Sheath – Annamaya Kosha – Physical Layer – Muscles and bones, then organs.
Muscles and Bones
_____
_____
_____

Organs
_____
_____

List physical direction cues in order. Reminder, "all yoga postures originate from the spine."
Would you teach this posture from the ground up or the spine out?
_____
_____
_____

Marianne's "-3 -2 -1 0 1 2 3"
List 3 ways to reduce this posture   List 3 ways to enhance this posture
_____   _____
_____   _____

List 3 Preparatory Postures   List 3 Subsequent Postures
_____   _____
_____   _____
_____   _____

Life Force Sheath – Pranamaya Kosha – Altered states of energetics through breath regulation.
How does your breath flow in this pose? Where do you get stuck? Where can you direct the breath?
_____
_____
_____

Mental Sheath – Manomaya Kosha – Our fluctuating mental and emotional layer.
How can this posture calm the fluctuations of the mind and emotions? Does the physical body interfere?
_____
_____
_____

Next Steps After Training, Pause and Reflect on –

Intellectual Sheath – Vijnanamaya Kosha – Self-study beyond thought, pure witness.
Have you ever experienced this place of pure space in this posture?

Bliss Sheath – Anandamaya Kosha – Love, Joy, Peace, Freedom
How does this posture help you move closer to the spiritualness of yoga?

Use the space below to draw this posture.

Pigeon Pose - Eka Pada Rajakapotasana - (aa-kah-pah-dah-rah-jah-cop-poh-tahs-anna)
(eka = one foot or leg) (raja = king) (kapota = pigeon)

Benefits

• **Stretches the thighs, groins, psoas, abdomen, chest, shoulders and neck - how?**

• **Opens the shoulders and chest - cautions?**

• **Stimulates the abdominal organs - how?**

Cautions

• **Knee injury - cautions?**

• **Ankle injury - cautions?**

• **Sacroiliac injury - cautions?**

• **Tight hips or thighs - cautions?**

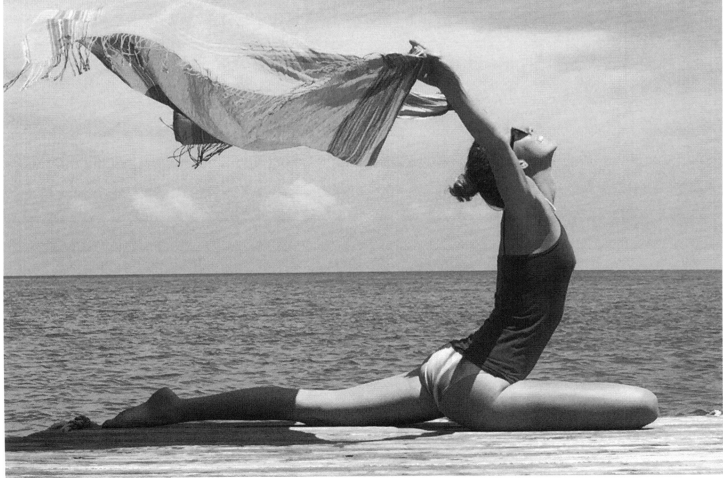

Anatomical Sheath – Annamaya Kosha – Physical Layer – Muscles and bones, then organs.
Muscles and Bones
_____
_____

Organs
_____
_____

List physical direction cues in order. Reminder, "all yoga postures originate from the spine."
Would you teach this posture from the ground up or the spine out?
_____
_____

Marianne's "-3 -2 -1 0 1 2 3"
List 3 ways to reduce this posture   List 3 ways to enhance this posture
_____   _____
_____   _____

List 3 Preparatory Postures   List 3 Subsequent Postures
_____   _____
_____   _____

Life Force Sheath – Pranamaya Kosha – Altered states of energetics through breath regulation.
How does your breath flow in this pose? Where do you get stuck? Where can you direct the breath?
_____
_____

Mental Sheath – Manomaya Kosha – Our fluctuating mental and emotional layer.
How can this posture calm the fluctuations of the mind and emotions? Does the physical body interfere?
_____
_____

Next Steps After Training, Pause and Reflect on –

Intellectual Sheath – Vijnanamaya Kosha – Self-study beyond thought, pure witness.
Have you ever experienced this place of pure space in this posture?

Bliss Sheath – Anandamaya Kosha – Love, Joy, Peace, Freedom
How does this posture help you move closer to the spiritualness of yoga?

Use the space below to draw this posture. ✍🖋🖋🖋

Plow Pose - Halasana - (hah-lahs-anna)
   (hala = plow)

Benefits

• Therapeutic for backache, headache, infertility, insomnia, sinusitis - cautions?

• Stimulates the abdominal organs and the thyroid gland - cautions?

• Helps relieve the symptoms of menopause - cautions?

• Stretches the shoulders and spine - cautions?

• Reduces stress and fatigue - cautions?

• Calms the brain - how?

Cautions

• High or low blood pressure - why?

• Neck injury - cautions?

• Menstruation - why?

• Diarrhea - why?

• Asthma - why?

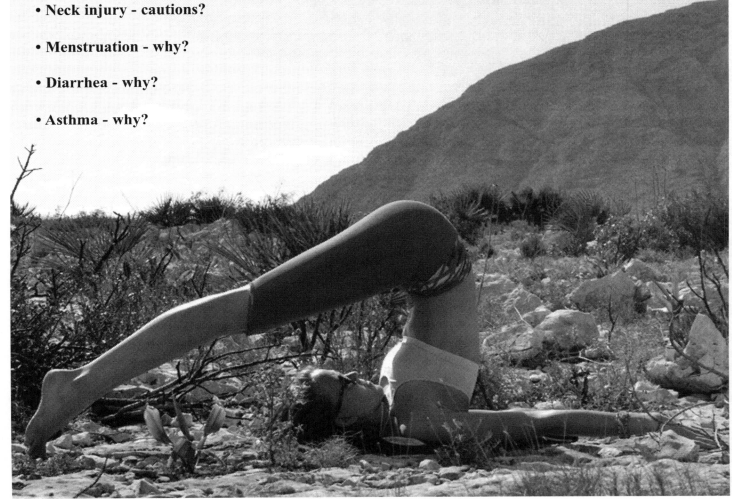

Anatomical Sheath – Annamaya Kosha – Physical Layer – Muscles and bones, then organs.
Muscles and Bones

_____

_____

Organs

_____

_____

List physical direction cues in order. Reminder, "all yoga postures originate from the spine."
Would you teach this posture from the ground up or the spine out?

_____

_____

Marianne's "-3 -2 -1 0 1 2 3"
List 3 ways to reduce this posture   List 3 ways to enhance this posture

_____   _____

_____   _____

List 3 Preparatory Postures   List 3 Subsequent Postures

_____   _____

_____   _____

Life Force Sheath – Pranamaya Kosha – Altered states of energetics through breath regulation.
How does your breath flow in this pose? Where do you get stuck? Where can you direct the breath?

_____

_____

Mental Sheath – Manomaya Kosha – Our fluctuating mental and emotional layer.
How can this posture calm the fluctuations of the mind and emotions? Does the physical body interfere?

_____

_____

Next Steps After Training, Pause and Reflect on –

Intellectual Sheath – Vijnanamaya Kosha – Self-study beyond thought, pure witness.
Have you ever experienced this place of pure space in this posture?

Bliss Sheath – Anandamaya Kosha – Love, Joy, Peace, Freedom
How does this posture help you move closer to the spiritualness of yoga?

Use the space below to draw this posture.

Extended Side Angle - Utthita Parsvakonasana - (oo-tee-tah parsh-vah-cone-ahs-anna)
(utthita = extended) (parsva = side, flank) (kona = angle)

Benefits

• Stretches the groins, spine, waist, chest, lungs, and shoulders - cautions?

• Strengthens and stretches the legs, knees, and ankles - how?

• Stimulates abdominal organs - cautions?

• Increases stamina - how?

Cautions

• Insomnia - why?

• Headache - why?

• Neck problems - why?

• High or low blood pressure - why?

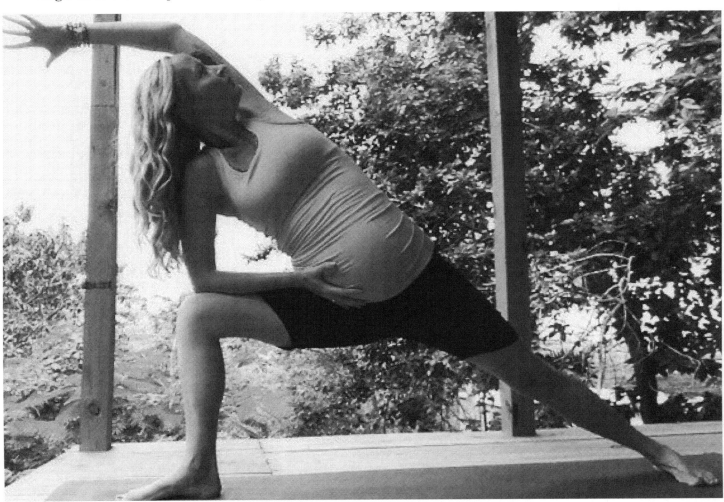

Anatomical Sheath – Annamaya Kosha – Physical Layer – Muscles and bones, then organs.
Muscles and Bones

_____

_____

Organs

_____

_____

List physical direction cues in order. Reminder, "all yoga postures originate from the spine."
Would you teach this posture from the ground up or the spine out?

_____

_____

Marianne's "-3 -2 -1 0 1 2 3"
List 3 ways to reduce this posture   List 3 ways to enhance this posture

_____   _____

_____   _____

List 3 Preparatory Postures   List 3 Subsequent Postures

_____   _____

_____   _____

Life Force Sheath – Pranamaya Kosha – Altered states of energetics through breath regulation.
How does your breath flow in this pose? Where do you get stuck? Where can you direct the breath?

_____

_____

Mental Sheath – Manomaya Kosha – Our fluctuating mental and emotional layer.
How can this posture calm the fluctuations of the mind and emotions? Does the physical body interfere?

_____

_____

Next Steps After Training, Pause and Reflect on –

Intellectual Sheath – Vijnanamaya Kosha – Self-study beyond thought, pure witness.
Have you ever experienced this place of pure space in this posture?

Bliss Sheath – Anandamaya Kosha – Love, Joy, Peace, Freedom
How does this posture help you move closer to the spiritualness of yoga?

Use the space below to draw this posture. ✍🖋🖋🖋

Seated Forward Fold Pose - Paschimottanasana - (posh-ee-moh-tan-ahs-anna)
(pashima = west) (uttana = intense stretch)

Benefits

• Traditional texts say that this pose increases appetite, reduces obesity, and cures diseases.

• Therapeutic for high blood pressure, infertility, insomnia, and sinusitis - why?

• Helps relieve the symptoms of menopause and menstrual discomfort - how?

• Calms the brain and helps relieve stress and mild depression - how?

• Soothes headache and anxiety and reduces fatigue - why?

• Stimulates the liver, kidneys, ovaries, and uterus - how?

• Stretches the spine, shoulders, hamstrings - cautions?

Cautions

• Asthma - why?

• Diarrhea - why?

• Back injury - why?

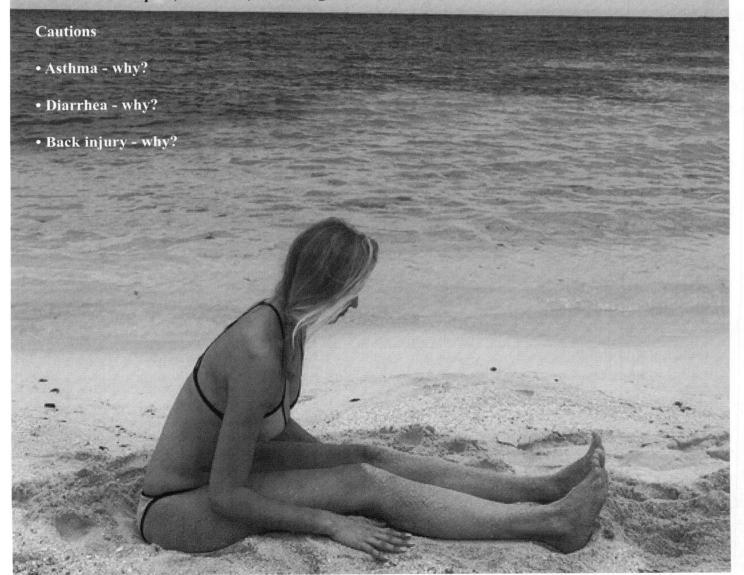

Anatomical Sheath – Annamaya Kosha – Physical Layer – Muscles and bones, then organs.
Muscles and Bones
_____
_____
_____
Organs
_____
_____

List physical direction cues in order. Reminder, "all yoga postures originate from the spine."
Would you teach this posture from the ground up or the spine out?
_____
_____
_____

Marianne's "-3 -2 -1 0 1 2 3"
List 3 ways to reduce this posture   List 3 ways to enhance this posture
_____   _____
_____   _____

List 3 Preparatory Postures   List 3 Subsequent Postures
_____   _____
_____   _____

Life Force Sheath – Pranamaya Kosha – Altered states of energetics through breath regulation.
How does your breath flow in this pose? Where do you get stuck? Where can you direct the breath?
_____
_____
_____

Mental Sheath – Manomaya Kosha – Our fluctuating mental and emotional layer.
How can this posture calm the fluctuations of the mind and emotions? Does the physical body interfere?
_____
_____
_____

Next Steps After Training, Pause and Reflect on –

Intellectual Sheath – Vijnanamaya Kosha – Self-study beyond thought, pure witness.
Have you ever experienced this place of pure space in this posture?

Bliss Sheath – Anandamaya Kosha – Love, Joy, Peace, Freedom
How does this posture help you move closer to the spiritualness of yoga?

Use the space below to draw this posture. ✍🖎🖎🖎

Staff Pose - Dandasana - (dahn-da-sana)
        (dand = staff)

Benefits

• Helps strengthen your back, hamstrings, feet and toes - cautions?

• A great overall posture - why?

Cautions

• Back injury - why?

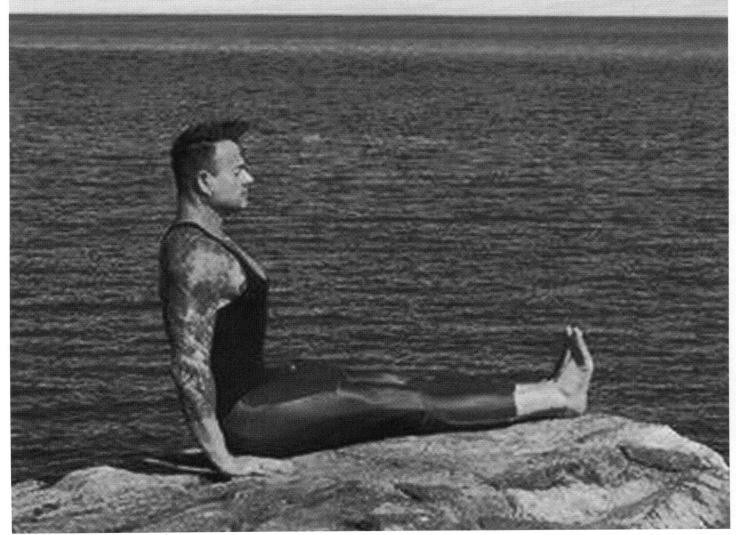

Anatomical Sheath – Annamaya Kosha – Physical Layer – Muscles and bones, then organs.
Muscles and Bones
_____
_____
_____

Organs
_____
_____
_____

List physical direction cues in order. Reminder, "all yoga postures originate from the spine."
Would you teach this posture from the ground up or the spine out?
_____
_____
_____

Marianne's "-3 -2 -1 0 1 2 3"

List 3 ways to reduce this posture   List 3 ways to enhance this posture
_____   _____
_____   _____
_____   _____

List 3 Preparatory Postures   List 3 Subsequent Postures
_____   _____
_____   _____
_____   _____

Life Force Sheath – Pranamaya Kosha – Altered states of energetics through breath regulation.
How does your breath flow in this pose? Where do you get stuck? Where can you direct the breath?
_____
_____
_____

Mental Sheath – Manomaya Kosha – Our fluctuating mental and emotional layer.
How can this posture calm the fluctuations of the mind and emotions? Does the physical body interfere?
_____
_____
_____

Next Steps After Training, Pause and Reflect on –

Intellectual Sheath – Vijnanamaya Kosha – Self-study beyond thought, pure witness.
Have you ever experienced this place of pure space in this posture?

Bliss Sheath – Anandamaya Kosha – Love, Joy, Peace, Freedom
How does this posture help you move closer to the spiritualness of yoga?

Use the space below to draw this posture.

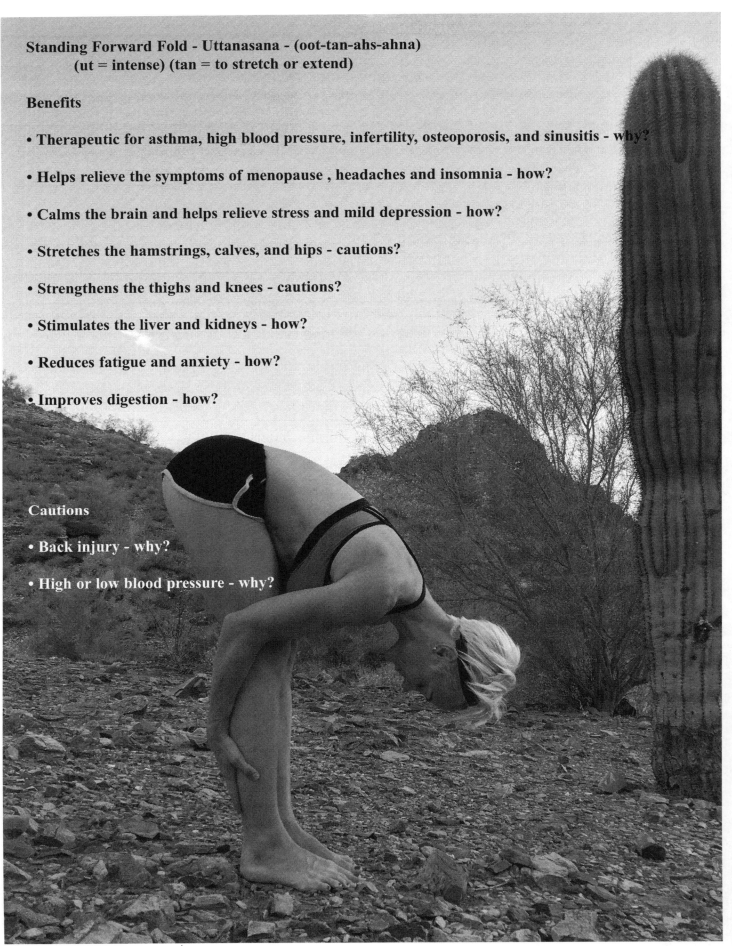

Standing Forward Fold - Uttanasana - (oot-tan-ahs-ahna)
       (ut = intense) (tan = to stretch or extend)

Benefits

• Therapeutic for asthma, high blood pressure, infertility, osteoporosis, and sinusitis - why?

• Helps relieve the symptoms of menopause , headaches and insomnia - how?

• Calms the brain and helps relieve stress and mild depression - how?

• Stretches the hamstrings, calves, and hips - cautions?

• Strengthens the thighs and knees - cautions?

• Stimulates the liver and kidneys - how?

• Reduces fatigue and anxiety - how?

• Improves digestion - how?

Cautions

• Back injury - why?

• High or low blood pressure - why?

Anatomical Sheath – Annamaya Kosha – Physical Layer – Muscles and bones, then organs.

Muscles and Bones

_____

_____

Organs

_____

_____

List physical direction cues in order. Reminder, "all yoga postures originate from the spine."
Would you teach this posture from the ground up or the spine out?

_____

_____

_____

Marianne's "-3 -2 -1 0 1 2 3"

List 3 ways to reduce this posture   List 3 ways to enhance this posture

_____   _____

_____   _____

_____   _____

List 3 Preparatory Postures   List 3 Subsequent Postures

_____   _____

_____   _____

_____   _____

Life Force Sheath – Pranamaya Kosha – Altered states of energetics through breath regulation.
How does your breath flow in this pose? Where do you get stuck? Where can you direct the breath?

_____

_____

_____

Mental Sheath – Manomaya Kosha – Our fluctuating mental and emotional layer.
How can this posture calm the fluctuations of the mind and emotions? Does the physical body interfere?

_____

_____

_____

Next Steps After Training, Pause and Reflect on –

Intellectual Sheath – Vijnanamaya Kosha – Self-study beyond thought, pure witness.
Have you ever experienced this place of pure space in this posture?

Bliss Sheath – Anandamaya Kosha – Love, Joy, Peace, Freedom
How does this posture help you move closer to the spiritualness of yoga?

Use the space below to draw this posture. ✍◯◯◯

Supported Shoulder Stand - Salamba Sarvangasana - (sah-lom-bah sar-van-gahs-anna)
(sa = with) (alamba = support) (sarva = all) (anga = limb

Benefits

• Stimulates the thyroid and prostate glands and abdominal organs - how?

• Calms the brain and helps relieve stress and mild depression - how?

• Therapeutic for asthma, infertility, and sinusitis - how?

• Helps relieve the symptoms of menopause - how?

• Reduces fatigue and alleviates insomnia - how?

• Stretches the shoulders and neck - cautions?

• Tones the legs and buttocks - how?

• Improves digestion - how?

Cautions

• Diarrhea - why?

• Headache - why?

• Menstruation - why?

• Neck injury - cautions?

• High or low blood pressure - why?

Anatomical Sheath – Annamaya Kosha – Physical Layer – Muscles and bones, then organs.
Muscles and Bones

_____

_____

_____

Organs

_____

_____

_____

List physical direction cues in order. Reminder, "all yoga postures originate from the spine."
Would you teach this posture from the ground up or the spine out?

_____

_____

_____

_____

Marianne's "-3 -2 -1 0 1 2 3"

List 3 ways to reduce this posture   List 3 ways to enhance this posture

_____   _____

_____   _____

_____   _____

List 3 Preparatory Postures   List 3 Subsequent Postures

_____   _____

_____   _____

_____   _____

Life Force Sheath – Pranamaya Kosha – Altered states of energetics through breath regulation.
How does your breath flow in this pose? Where do you get stuck? Where can you direct the breath?

_____

_____

_____

Mental Sheath – Manomaya Kosha – Our fluctuating mental and emotional layer.
How can this posture calm the fluctuations of the mind and emotions? Does the physical body interfere?

_____

_____

_____

Next Steps After Training, Pause and Reflect on –

Intellectual Sheath – Vijnanamaya Kosha – Self-study beyond thought, pure witness.
Have you ever experienced this place of pure space in this posture?

Bliss Sheath – Anandamaya Kosha – Love, Joy, Peace, Freedom
How does this posture help you move closer to the spiritualness of yoga?

Use the space below to draw this posture.

Tree Pose - Vrksasana - (vrik-shahs-anna)
   (vrksa = tree)

Benefits

• **Stretches the groins and inner thighs, chest and shoulders - cautions?**

• **Brings ease to sciatica pain and reduces flat feet- how?**

• **Strengthens thighs, calves, ankles, and spine - how?**

• **Relieves anxiety and fatigue - why?**

• **Improves sense of balance - how?**

Cautions

• **High or low blood pressure- why?**

• **Insomnia - why?**

• **Headache - why?**

Anatomical Sheath – Annamaya Kosha – Physical Layer – Muscles and bones, then organs.
Muscles and Bones

_____

_____

Organs

_____

_____

List physical direction cues in order. Reminder, "all yoga postures originate from the spine."
Would you teach this posture from the ground up or the spine out?

_____

_____

Marianne's "-3 -2 -1 0 1 2 3"
List 3 ways to reduce this posture   List 3 ways to enhance this posture

_____   _____

_____   _____

List 3 Preparatory Postures   List 3 Subsequent Postures

_____   _____

_____   _____

Life Force Sheath – Pranamaya Kosha – Altered states of energetics through breath regulation.
How does your breath flow in this pose? Where do you get stuck? Where can you direct the breath?

_____

_____

_____

Mental Sheath – Manomaya Kosha – Our fluctuating mental and emotional layer.
How can this posture calm the fluctuations of the mind and emotions? Does the physical body interfere?

_____

_____

_____

Next Steps After Training, Pause and Reflect on –

Intellectual Sheath – Vijnanamaya Kosha – Self-study beyond thought, pure witness.
Have you ever experienced this place of pure space in this posture?

Bliss Sheath – Anandamaya Kosha – Love, Joy, Peace, Freedom
How does this posture help you move closer to the spiritualness of yoga?

Use the space below to draw this posture. ✎✐✐✐

Extended Triangle - Utthita Trikonasana - (oo-tee-tah trik-cone-ahs-anna)
        (utthita = extended) (trikona = three angle or triangle)

Benefits

• **Stretches the hips, groins, hamstrings, and calves; shoulders, chest, and spine - cautions?**

• **Therapeutic for anxiety, flat feet, infertility, neck pain, osteoporosis, and sciatica - how?**

• **Relieves backache, especially through second trimester of pregnancy - cautions?**

• **Stretches and strengthens the thighs, knees, and ankles - cautions?**

• **Helps relieve the symptoms of menopause - how?**

• **Stimulates the abdominal organs - how?**

• **Helps relieve stress - how?**

• **Improves digestion - why?**

Cautions

• **Diarrhea - why?**

• **Headache - why?**

• **Neck problems - why?**

• **Heart condition - why?**

• **High or low blood pressure - why?**

Anatomical Sheath – Annamaya Kosha – Physical Layer – Muscles and bones, then organs.
Muscles and Bones

_____
_____
_____

Organs

_____
_____

List physical direction cues in order. Reminder, "all yoga postures originate from the spine."
Would you teach this posture from the ground up or the spine out?

_____
_____
_____

Marianne's "-3 -2 -1 0 1 2 3"
List 3 ways to reduce this posture   List 3 ways to enhance this posture

_____   _____
_____   _____
_____   _____

List 3 Preparatory Postures   List 3 Subsequent Postures

_____   _____
_____   _____
_____   _____

Life Force Sheath – Pranamaya Kosha – Altered states of energetics through breath regulation.
How does your breath flow in this pose? Where do you get stuck? Where can you direct the breath?

_____
_____
_____

Mental Sheath – Manomaya Kosha – Our fluctuating mental and emotional layer.
How can this posture calm the fluctuations of the mind and emotions? Does the physical body interfere?

_____
_____
_____

Next Steps After Training, Pause and Reflect on –

Intellectual Sheath – Vijnanamaya Kosha – Self-study beyond thought, pure witness.
Have you ever experienced this place of pure space in this posture?

Bliss Sheath – Anandamaya Kosha – Love, Joy, Peace, Freedom
How does this posture help you move closer to the spiritualness of yoga?

Use the space below to draw this posture. ✍🍃🍃🍃

Upward Bow Pose - Urdhva Dhanurasana - (oord-vah don-your-ahs-anna)
   (urdhva = upward) (dhanu = bow)

Benefits

• **Strengthens the arms and wrists, legs, buttocks, abdomen, and spine - how?**

• **Therapeutic for asthma, back pain, infertility, and osteoporosis - how?**

• **Increases energy and counteracts depression - how?**

• **Stimulates the thyroid and pituitary - how?**

• **Stretches the chest and lungs - how?**

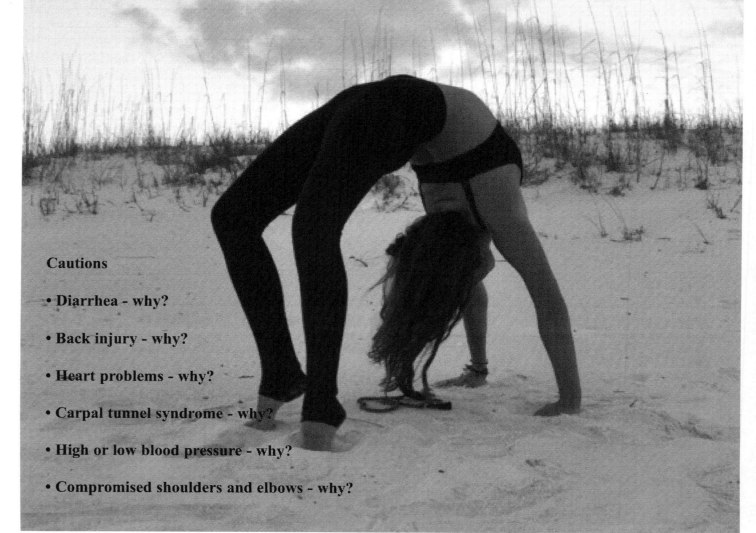

Cautions

• **Diarrhea - why?**

• **Back injury - why?**

• **Heart problems - why?**

• **Carpal tunnel syndrome - why?**

• **High or low blood pressure - why?**

• **Compromised shoulders and elbows - why?**

Anatomical Sheath – Annamaya Kosha – Physical Layer – Muscles and bones, then organs.
Muscles and Bones

_____

_____

Organs

_____

_____

List physical direction cues in order. Reminder, "all yoga postures originate from the spine."
Would you teach this posture from the ground up or the spine out?

_____

_____

_____

Marianne's "-3 -2 -1 0 1 2 3"
List 3 ways to reduce this posture   List 3 ways to enhance this posture

_____   _____

_____   _____

_____   _____

List 3 Preparatory Postures   List 3 Subsequent Postures

_____   _____

_____   _____

_____   _____

Life Force Sheath – Pranamaya Kosha – Altered states of energetics through breath regulation.
How does your breath flow in this pose? Where do you get stuck? Where can you direct the breath?

_____

_____

_____

Mental Sheath – Manomaya Kosha – Our fluctuating mental and emotional layer.
How can this posture calm the fluctuations of the mind and emotions? Does the physical body interfere?

_____

_____

_____

Next Steps After Training, Pause and Reflect on –

Intellectual Sheath – Vijnanamaya Kosha – Self-study beyond thought, pure witness.
Have you ever experienced this place of pure space in this posture?

Bliss Sheath – Anandamaya Kosha – Love, Joy, Peace, Freedom
How does this posture help you move closer to the spiritualness of yoga?

Use the space below to draw this posture.

Warrior One - Virabhadrasana One - (veer-ah-bah-drahs-anna)
        (veer = strong)

Benefits

• **Strengthens the shoulders and arms, and the muscles of the back - how?**

• **Stretches the chest and lungs, shoulders and neck, belly, groins - how?**

• **Strengthens and stretches the thighs, calves, and ankles - how?**

Cautions

• **Heart problems - why?**

• **Neck problems - why?**

• **Shoulder problems - why?**

• **High or low blood pressure - why?**

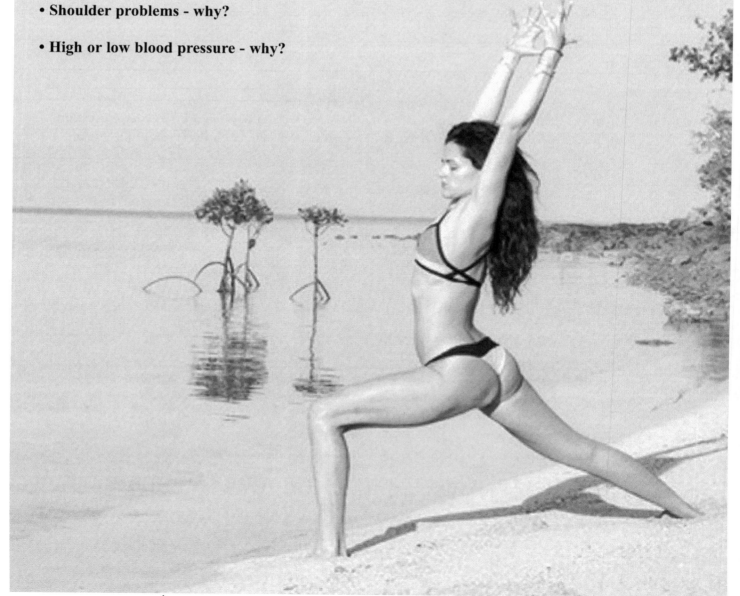

Anatomical Sheath – Annamaya Kosha – Physical Layer – Muscles and bones, then organs.
Muscles and Bones

_____
_____

Organs

_____
_____

List physical direction cues in order. Reminder, "all yoga postures originate from the spine."
Would you teach this posture from the ground up or the spine out?

_____
_____
_____

Marianne's "-3 -2 -1 0 1 2 3"
List 3 ways to reduce this posture   List 3 ways to enhance this posture

_____   _____
_____   _____
_____   _____

List 3 Preparatory Postures   List 3 Subsequent Postures

_____   _____
_____   _____
_____   _____

Life Force Sheath – Pranamaya Kosha – Altered states of energetics through breath regulation.
How does your breath flow in this pose? Where do you get stuck? Where can you direct the breath?

_____
_____
_____

Mental Sheath – Manomaya Kosha – Our fluctuating mental and emotional layer.
How can this posture calm the fluctuations of the mind and emotions? Does the physical body interfere?

_____
_____
_____

Next Steps After Training, Pause and Reflect on –

Intellectual Sheath – Vijnanamaya Kosha – Self-study beyond thought, pure witness.
Have you ever experienced this place of pure space in this posture?

Bliss Sheath – Anandamaya Kosha – Love, Joy, Peace, Freedom
How does this posture help you move closer to the spiritualness of yoga?

Use the space below to draw this posture. ✍✎✎✎

SAVASANA

Corpse Pose – Savasana

Savasana is the mac daddy of all relaxation postures and the hardest to practice. Mental happiness is total relaxation! It is not easy to turn our mind inward. Corpse pose should conclude both your asana and your pranayama practices. Abdominal breathing is conscious breath work best done in corpse pose. Inhale slowly and deeply, feeling the torso rise on the inhale. Slowly and deeply exhale, feeling the torso relax on the exhale. Become aware of your diaphragm. Understand that it is a muscle between the lungs and stomach. Feel the energy of your breath from the nose to the throat to the lungs to the belly to the pelvis and back out the same path.

Savasana is the beginning of a bandha practice. Asanas are practiced to become familiar with our bodies and aware of our lifestyles. A bandha practice is very much like practicing Tai Chi. Bandhas are like space – one requires walls or boundaries to define the space. You should only practice bandha work after you have established a breath ratio and can hold that breathe ratio for 12 breaths. For most practitioners, bandha work should only be practiced during savasana and pranayama – not during an asana practice.

While in corpse pose, teachers can check a student's physical alignment by sitting at the head. Observe the head position relative to the shoulders; it is common for the head to be tilted or turned to one side or the other. The teacher should gently cradle the head in his/her hands and draw the base of the skull away from the back of the neck – lengthening the shorter side of the neck – so that both ears are equidistant from the shoulders. The teacher can then lower the head to the floor, making sure that the tip of the nose points directly toward the ceiling.

Benefits
• Calms the brain and helps relieve stress and mild depression. How?

• Relaxes the body. Why?

• Reduces headache, fatigue and insomnia. How?

• Helps to lower blood pressure. How?

Cautions
• Savasana should be modified for students experiencing back discomfort. Why?

• Savasana should be modified for students who are pregnant. Why?

BANDHAS

STOP ACTING SO SMALL. YOU ARE THE UNIVERSE IN ECSTATIC MOTION ~ RUMI

The Bandhas – Jalandhara, Uddiyana, Mula

Also known as body locks or pumps and valves, bandhas are a combination of muscle contraction and creation of space. Designed to change blood circulation and flow of energy, the bandhas rechannel tension, helping to raise consciousness and healing. You have a body and a mind and a spirit. What rules the body is not what rules the mind and spirit. Along with a strong physical practice, you need a strong mental and spiritual practice. Like Gandhi, practice meditation without violence and ego. Pull into yourself. Keep arranging yourself so that you are grounded and you spiral up from the earth. Props are good for pranayama, use what is needed to be physically comfortable with a straight spine and closed eyes. At the age of 78, Iyengar considered himself a beginner, always saying that all we need is Tadasana and Savasana. However, we need all the other poses to discover all the areas of your body. There is a difference between doing the pose, feeling the pose, and using the pose to wake up consciousness. Be the observer in action. The more skilled in observation, the more skilled in action. Skillful action allows for peace inside; with unskillful action, there is less peace inside. Learn to practice like a musician. When you get to difficult parts, slow down to study. Learn to go to the space around the bandhas, feel the creation of that space open up and the release of vibrations in the entire body.

Neck Lock – Jalandhara Bandha

The jalandhara bandha helps to depressurize the head and throat areas, including the sense organs and crown, third eye and throat chakras.

Diaphragm Lock – Uddiyana Bandha

The uddiyana bandha or diaphragm lock is an almost automatic side-effect of a strong mula bandha. The uddiyana bandha action is an upward movement. The low belly and navel area pull in and up, firming the abdomen and drawing the breath up into the rib cage, chest and lungs. This action brings energy, affecting the sympathetic nervous system and removal of stress. The diaphragm moves freely and, with practice, the uddiyana bandha increases lung capacity.

Root Lock – Mula Bandha

The mula bandha or root lock is a traditional hatha yoga energy producing practice. By actively engaging the mula bandha, energy is intensified at the base of the spine. The area between anus and scrotum or clitoris is contracted; the perineal muscle group stimulates the fibers that emerge from base of spinal column.

MEDITATION

YOU SHOULD SIT IN MEDITATION FOR TWENTY MINUTES EVERY DAY, UNLESS YOU ARE BUSY, THEN YOU SHOULD SIT FOR AN HOUR. ~ OLD ZEN ADAGE

Why Meditate

Meditation means being "pleasantly anchored in the present moment." With our hectic lifestyles, stress is a strong contributor to heart disease and high blood pressure. It is important to learn to relax our mind and body. Meditation is easy to incorporate into our lives. Scientists study it, doctors recommend it, and millions of people all over the world practice it daily. Meditation can help us develop hidden talents that we had forgotten we possess. Through meditation, we can achieve more with less effort, with a more alert brain and relaxed heart. It refreshes us completely and gets us ready for another batch of work. Meditation helps block out distractions that may come our way.

All energy moves toward joy. There are many types of meditation, some ancient, some newer; different styles, systems, names, traditions, lineages and religions. Among them all is a commonality of focus. Meditation is the connection between mind and body to help achieve specific developmental goals. Meditation is particularly good in reducing stress that you encounter and develop in everyday life. When we detach from stress, it can help form the basis of enabling personal growth, often in a creative way. When you decide to make meditation a regular part of your life, decide which type is best for you.

Meditation Guidelines

Consistency – Set aside time daily, either before you start your day and/or just before bed. Allow fiffteen minutes for each meditation session to start. With consistency this may become longer. On days with less formal schedules, try meditate for longer periods of time. One hour would be optimal to enter deeper states of meditation. Success in meditation arises from consistency and regularity of your practice.

Create a Familiar Space – While there are countless ways to meditate on the go, creating a sacred space in your home or office to meditate is best for serious beginners. Create an altar with inspirational items, symbols, candles, incense.

Assume a Comfortable Position – You do not need to sit on the floor; you can use a chair. The key is to keep a tall spine. Learn how to sit and options for placement of your hands.

Utilize Accessories to Help Maintain Your Focus at First – But remember, as wonderful as mala beads, candles, even apps, etc., are, your breath is all you really need.

Rituals – Rituals have deep meaning and play a key role in a meditation practice. Like a child sleeping with a favorite toy, rituals can calm the mind and bring a sense of safety and familiarity. It is important to ground yourself after meditation. Take time to feel your feet, body and active mind. Drink tea. Start with slow movements in all limbs, eyes and face to activate the nerve pathways that slow down during intense meditation.

Types of Meditation Practices

Concentration – complete focus on only one object.

Examples –
• Rock – can represent grounding, the earth, stability of form
• Flower – can represent beauty, color, form, renewal, growth
• Flame – can represent movement, transformation, action, the sun
• Saint – can represent God, love, transcendence
• Nothing – can represent release of all thought, mindfulness

Sensation – focused on simple thoughts in rhythm with movement – while walking, or during an inhalation or exhalation add thoughts such as –
• I – Am
• Seek – That
• Right – Now
• Just – Be

Love–Joy–Peace – focused on Higher states of loving kindness – compassion – happiness – acceptance – gratitude – joy – or healing to ourselves, our loved ones, and even those who we don't like.

Mantra – In Sanskrit, mantra means "mind instrument." To us, it means a sound, syllable or group of sounds. Mantra repetition is an ancient meditation technique extensively used in Tibet and India. Mantra involves repeating a sentence or group of words that have a phonetic significance. Mantra is sound – vibrations that exist in everything in the universe. When water flows, the gurgling sound it makes is mantra. When wind blows through the trees, the rustling sound it produces is mantra. When we walk on the earth, our footsteps produce sound and that, too, is mantra. Sound has enormous power. In fact, it has the power to create an entire universe.

In India, the belief was the sound at the beginning of creation of the universe was Om or Aum. A mantra is no ordinary combination of syllables, but a living force that we experience for ourselves.

The name of God is not different from God. Mantra has been called the sound-body of God. It is God in the form of sound. In the Bhagavad Gita, Lord Krishna says, "Among rituals, I am the ritual of mantra repetition." While other techniques are means of attaining God, mantra is God's very being. That is why it is so easy to experience God by repeating the mantra. Mantra meditation is repetition, which create sound vibrations, that awake the love of God in our hearts and mind.

Aum represents the union of the three Gods. Aum is said to be the primordial sound that was present at the creation of the universe. It is the original sound that contains all other sounds, all words, all languages and all mantras.

• A (ahh) represents Brahma – the creator of all existence.
• U (uhh) represents Vishnu – the preserver of existing creation.
• M (mmm) represents Shiva – the destroyer and final part of the cycle of existence.

Benefits of Meditation

Meditation has been used for centuries in cultures all over the world as a method for relaxation, improving health, and finding mental clarity. For as little as 10 minutes a day, it can bring about significant positive changes – a solitary act that requires no outside influence or money.

Spiritually

- Deepens religious/spiritual devotion and understanding.
- Offers an opportunity to develop a deeper understanding of oneself.
- Allows an individual to feel a sense of connection to everything and everyone – increasing one's personal capacity for love and acceptance.

Mentally

- Develops emotional maturity as one learns to be calm in the face of drama.
- Increases the release of serotonin in the brain, a chemical that improves mood and naturally makes one feel good.
- Increases self-confidence.
- Helps prevent panic attacks in those who suffer from anxiety disorders.
- Helps improve memory and the ability to learn new things.
- Enables one to see the big picture in order to solve complex problems.
- Reduces aggressive behavior in individuals.
- Helps with the process required to break bad habits and addictions such as smoking, drinking and drugs.
- Slows down racing thoughts that often keep people distracted and awake at night.
- Improves patience when others would become annoyed.
- Keeps mental faculties sharp and slows down the effects of age on the brain.
- Shifts brain activity to less stress-prone areas of the brain, decreasing the negative effects of mild stress, depression and anxiety.
- Helps one to release negative emotions rather than allowing them to become one's focus.
- Provides clarity, helps to simplify one's life, quieting inner turmoil or recognizing the need for fewer material goods in life.
- Increases energy levels.
- Increases creative output by improving communication between left and right hemispheres with less clutter and better focus in new directions.
- Can be used in conjunction with other forms of medicine or therapy to enhance physical and mental outcomes.
- Improves one's ability to "live in the present," rather than always fretting over future desires or past regrets.
- Improves the ability to recognize one's own thought patterns, allowing for self-reflection, acknowledgement and even change.
- Removes obstacles preventing individuals from succeeding, brings clarity of thought to make appropriate changes on the path to success.
- Hand-eye coordination increases within individuals who practice meditation.
- Breath is the secret to "mindfulness."

Physically

- Improves the flow of oxygen to the brain, bringing clearer thinking and better reasoning skills.
- Improves blood flow to the muscles – this helps with physical stamina. Exercise more easily and for longer periods of time.
- Decreases muscle tension, resulting not only in better relaxation, but also a lower likelihood of sustaining an injury.
- Slows respiration, decreases asthma attacks and other breathing issues.
- Relaxes the nervous system, leading to a decrease in multiple stress-induced reactions.
- Lowers the heart rate to healthier levels. Helps to normalize blood pressure.
- Can reduce risk of heart disease.
- Decreases physical pain, especially for chronic pain sufferers.
- Lessens the severity of physical and emotional symptoms of pre-menstrual syndrome and other stress factors.
- Helps increase the overall goals of weight-loss programs due to a lowering of cortisol, as well as other factors.
- Restores the body to a calm state once the flight or fight response has been triggered by an environmental stressor.
- Boosts the immune system to help ward off physical ailments and diseases.
- Strengthens the digestive system for improved overall health and wellness of the body.

IF YOU WANT TO LIVE LIFE FREE

TAKE YOUR TIME

GO SLOWLY

DO FEW THINGS

BUT DO THEM WELL ·

SIMPLE JOYS ARE HOLY

~ FRANCIS OF ASSISI

FOR IN THE END

WE WILL CONSERVE

ONLY WHAT WE LOVE

WE WILL LOVE

ONLY WHAT WE UNDERSTAND

WE WILL UNDERSTAND

ONLY WHAT WE LEARN

~ MARIANNE WELLS

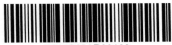
Made in the USA
Columbia, SC
18 September 2018